Occupational Therapy in Forensic Psychiatry: Role Development and Schizophrenia

Occupational Therapy in Forensic Psychiatry: Role Development and Schizophrenia has been co-published simultaneously as *Occupational Therapy in Mental Health*, Volume 20, Numbers 3/4 2004.

D1394451

Occupational Therapy in Mental Health Monographic "Separates"

Below is a list of "separates," which in serials librarianship means a special issue simultaneously published as a special journal issue or double-issue _and_ as a "separate" hardbound monograph. (This is a format which we also call a "DocuSerial.")

"Separates" are published because specialized libraries or professionals may wish to purchase a specific thematic issue by itself in a format which can be separately cataloged and shelved, as opposed to purchasing the journal on an on-going basis. Faculty members may also more easily consider a "separate" for classroom adoption.

"Separates" are carefully classified separately with the major book jobbers so that the journal tie-in can be noted on new book order slips to avoid duplicate purchasing.

You may wish to visit Haworth's website at . . .

http://www.HaworthPress.com

. . . to search our online catalog for complete tables of contents of these separates and related publications.

You may also call 1-800-HAWORTH (outside US/Canada: 607-722-5857), or Fax 1-800-895-0582 (outside US/Canada: 607-771-0012), or e-mail at:

docdelivery@haworthpress.com

Occupational Therapy in Forensic Psychiatry: Role Development and Schizophrenia, by Victoria P. Schindler, PhD, OTR (Vol. 20, No. 3/4, 2004). _"DR. SCHINDLER HAS ANSWERED OUR PROFESSION'S CALL for more evidence-based practice by using both basic and applied scientific inquiry to investigate how individuals diagnosed with schizophrenia can develop meaningful life roles while in a maximum-security psychiatric facility. Her findings clearly demonstrate the value of focusing intervention on helping clients pursue meaningful occupations through role development, rather than simply focusing on individual components of treatment." (Laurie Knis-Matthews, OT, MA, Assistant Professor, Kean University)_

Surviving 9/11: Impact and Experiences of Occupational Therapy Practitioners, edited by Pat Precin, MS, OTR/L (Vol. 19, No. 3/4, 2003). _Analyzes the many roles occupational therapy practitioners played during the tragic events of 9/11; examines new therapeutic practices developed because of the terrorist attacks._

An Ethnographic Study of Mental Health Treatment and Outcomes: Doing What Works, by Fran Babiss, PhD, OTR/L (Vol. 18, No. 3/4, 2002). _"All mental health clinicians and scholars will find this book INSIGHTFUL AND PROVOCATIVE. This book contains more than a description of three women living with anorexia nervosa: the rich qualitative data captures their pain and their struggles with daily life to survive." (Jim Hinojosa, PhD, OT, FAOTA, Professor and Chair, Department of Occupational Therapy, New York University)_

Recovery and Wellness: Models of Hope and Empowerment for People with Mental Illness, edited by Catana Brown, PhD, OTR/L, FAOTA (Vol. 17, No. 3/4, 2001). _Provides guidelines for incorporating wellness and recovery principles into mental health services using the Recovery Model._

Domestic Abuse Across the Lifespan: The Role of Occupational Therapy, by Christine A. Helfrich, PhD, OTR/L (Vol. 16, No. 3/4, 2001). _"For those occupational therapists who view themselves as holistic service providers, this book is a must-read. . . . Includes examples, studies, and research results." (Linda T. Learneard, OTR/L, President, Occupational Therapy Consultation and Rehabilitation Services, Inc.)_

Brain Injury and Gender Role Strain: Rebuilding Adult Lifestyles After Injury, by Sharon A. Gutman, PhD, OTR (Vol. 15, No. 3/4, 2000). _"Dr. Gutman has developed an innovative target setting and treatment planning protocol that focuses the therapist on the key areas of concern. I highly recommend this book to therapists who work with clients in the post-acute period of recovery from TBI." (Gordon Muir Giles, MA, Dip COT, OTR, Director of Neurobehavioral Services, Crestwood Behavioral Health, Inc., and Assistant Professor, Samuel Merritt College, Oakland, California)_

New Frontiers in Psychosocial Occupational Therapy, edited by Anne Hiller Scott, PhD, OTR, FAOTA (Vol. 14, No. 1/2, 1998). *"Speaks a clear message about mental health practice in occupational therapy, shattering old visions of practice to insights about empowerment and advocacy." (Sharan L. Schwartzberg, EdD, OTR, FAOTA, Professor and Chair, Boston School of Occupational Therapy, Tufts University)*

Evaluation and Treatment of the Psychogeriatric Patient, edited by Diane Gibson, MS, OTR (Vol. 10, No. 3, 1991). *"Occupational therapists everywhere, learners and sophisticates alike, and in-hospital and out-patient areas as well as home-bound and home-active, would enjoy and profit from this exposition as much as I did." (American Association of Psychiatric Administrators)*

Student Recruitment in Psychosocial Occupational Therapy: Intergenerational Approaches, edited by Susan Haiman (Vol. 10, No. 1, 1990). *"Can serve to enlighten both academics and clinicians as to their roles in attracting students to become practitioners in mental health settings. Each article could well serve as a catalyst for discussion in the classroom or clinic." (Canadian Journal of Occupational Therapy)*

Group Protocols: A Psychosocial Compendium, edited by Susan Haiman (Vol. 9, No. 4, 1990). *"Presents succinct protocols for a wide range of groups that are typically run by activities therapists, vocational counselors, art therapists, and other mental health professionals." (International Journal of Group Psychotherapy)*

Instrument Development in Occupational Therapy, edited by Janet Hawkins Watts and Chestina Brollier (Vol. 8, No. 4, 1989). *Examines content and concurrent validity and development of the Assessment of Occupational Functioning (AOF), and carefully compares the AOF with a similar instrument, the Occupational Case Analysis Interview and Rating Scale (OCAIRS), to discover the similarities and strengths of these instruments.*

Group Process and Structure in Psychosocial Occupational Therapy, edited by Diane Gibson, MS, OTR (Vol. 8, No. 3, 1989). *Highly skilled professionals examine the important concepts of group therapy to help build cohesive, safe groups.*

Treatment of Substance Abuse: Psychosocial Occupational Therapy Approaches, edited by Diane Gibson, MS, OTR (Vol. 8, No. 2, 1989). *A unique overview of contemporary assessment and rehabilitation of alcohol and chemical dependent substance abusers.*

The Development of Standardized Clinical Evaluations in Mental Health, Principal Investigator: Noomi Katz, PhD, OTR; edited by Claudia Kay Allen, MA, OTR, FAOTA; Commentator: Janice P. Burke, MA, OTR, FAOTA (Vol. 8, No. 1, 1988). *"Contains a collection of research-based articles encompassing several evaluations that can be used by occupational therapists practicing in mental health." (American Journal of Occupational Therapy)*

Evaluation and Treatment of Adolescents and Children, edited by Diane Gibson, MS, OTR (Vol. 7, No. 2, 1987). *Experts share research results and practices that have proven successful in helping young people who suffer from psychiatric and medical disorders.*

Treatment of the Chronic Schizophrenic Patient, edited by Diane Gibson, MS, OTR (Vol. 6, No. 2, 1986). *"Reflect[s] creative and fresh concepts of current treatment for the chronically mentally ill. . . . Recommended for the therapist practicing in psychiatry." (Canadian Journal of Occupational Therapy)*

The Evaluation and Treatment of Eating Disorders, edited by Diane Gibson, MS, OTR (Vol. 6, No. 1, 1986). *"A wealth of information. . . . Covers the subject thoroughly. . . . This book, well-conceived and well-written, is recommended not only for clinicians working with clients with anorexia nervosa and bulimia but for all therapists who wish to become acquainted with the subject of eating disorders in general." (Library Journal)*

Philosophical and Historical Roots of Occupational Therapy, edited by Karen Diasio Serrett (Vol. 5, No. 3, 1985). *"Recommended as an easy-to-get-through background read for occupational therapists and for generalists wishing a fuller acquaintance with the backdrop of occupational therapy." (Rehabilitation Literature)*

Short-Term Treatment in Occupational Therapy, edited by Diane Gibson, MS, OTR, and Kathy Kaplan, MS, OTR (Vol. 4, No. 3, 1984). *"Thought provoking and relevant to various issues facing OTs in a short term inpatient psychiatric setting. . . . Very readable . . . concise, well-written, and stimulating." (Canadian Journal of Occupational Therapy)*

SCORE: Solving Community Obstacles and Restoring Employment, by Lynn Wechsler Kramer, MS, OTR (Vol. 4, No. 1, 1984). *"This needed book is an effective instrument for occupational therapists wanting to 'teach employable handicapped how to obtain a job in a competitive (labor) market.' Very relevant to professional practice . . . a useful how-to instrument."* (The American Journal of Occupational Therapy)

Occupational Therapy with Borderline Patients, edited by Diane Gibson, MS, OTR (Vol. 3, No. 3, 1983). *"Offers clinicians an opportunity to review current theoretical concepts, management, and design of activity groups for this population. Well written . . . provides good reference lists and well-developed discussions."* (The American Journal of Occupational Therapy)

Psychiatric Occupational Therapy in the Army, edited by LTC Paul D. Ellsworth, MPH, OTR, FAOTA, and Diane Gibson, MS, OTR (Vol. 3, No. 2, 1983). *This unique volume focuses on the historical contributions, current trends, and future directions of army occupational therapists practicing in the military mental health arena.*

Occupational Therapy in Forensic Psychiatry: Role Development and Schizophrenia

Victoria P. Schindler, PhD, OTR

Occupational Therapy in Forensic Psychiatry: Role Development and Schizophrenia has been co-published simultaneously as *Occupational Therapy in Mental Health*, Volume 20, Numbers 3/4 2004.

The Haworth Press, Inc.

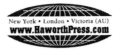

New York • London • Victoria (AU)
www.HaworthPress.com

Occupational Therapy in Forensic Psychiatry: Role Development and Schizophrenia has been co-published simultaneously as *Occupational Therapy in Mental Health*™, Volume 20, Numbers 3/4 2004.

Cover design by Jennifer Gaska

Library of Congress Cataloging-in-Publication Data

Schindler, Victoria P.
Occupational therapy in forensic psychiatry : role development and schizophrenia / Victoria P. Schindler.
     p. ; cm.
     "Co-published simultaneously as Occupational therapy in mental health, Volume 20, Numbers 3/4 2004."
     Includes bibliographical references and index.
     ISBN 0-7890-2124-2 (hard cover : alk. paper) – ISBN 0-7890-2125-0 (soft cover : alk. paper)
     1. Schizophrenics–Rehabilitation. 2. Social role. 3. Occupational therapy. 4. Forensic psychiatry.
     [DNLM: 1. Schizophrenia–rehabilitation–Case Reports. 2. Forensic Psychiatry–methods–Case Reports. 3. Occupational Therapy–methods–Case Reports. 4. Social Adjustment–Case Reports. 5. Treatment Outcome–Case Reports. WM 203 S336o 2004] I. Occupational therapy in mental health. II. Title.
RC514.S333 2004
616.89'806–dc22
                                                   2004017178

Indexing, Abstracting & Website/Internet Coverage

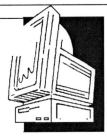

This section provides you with a list of major indexing & abstracting services and other tools for bibliographic access. That is to say, each service began covering this periodical during the year noted in the right column. Most Websites which are listed below have indicated that they will either post, disseminate; compile, archive, cite or alert their own Website users with research-based content from this work. (This list is as current as the copyright date of this publication.)

Abstracting, Website/Indexing Coverage . . . . Year When Coverage Began

- *Abstracts in Social Gerontology: Current Literature on Aging* **1993**

- *Alzheimer's Disease Education & Referral Center (ADEAR)* **1997**

- *Biosciences Information Service of Biological Abstracts (BIOSIS), a centralized source of life science information* *<http://www.biosis.org>* **1982**

- *Brandon/Hill Selected List of Journals in Allied Health Sciences* *<http://www.mssm.edu/library/brandon-hill/>* **2000**

- *Business Source Corporate: coverage of nearly 3,350 quality magazines and journals; designed to meet the diverse information needs of corporations; EBSCO Publishing* *<http://www.epnet.com/corporate/bsourcecorp.asp>* **2003**

- *CINAHL (Cumulative Index to Nursing & Allied Health Literature), in print, EBSCO, and SilverPlatter, Data-Star, and PaperChase. (Support materials include Subject Heading List, Database Search Guide, and instructional video.)* *<http://www.cinahl.com>* **1980**

- *Developmental Medicine & Child Neurology* **1994**

(continued)

- *EMBASE/Excerpta Medica Secondary Publishing Division. Included in newsletters, review journals, major reference works, magazines & abstract journals <http://www.elsevier.nl>* 1980
- *e-psyche, LLC <http://www.e-psyche.net>* 2000
- *Exceptional Child Education Resources (ECER) (CD/ROM from SilverPlatter and hard copy) <http://www.ericec.org/ecer-db.html>* 1993
- *Excerpta Medica .... see EMBASE* 1980
- *Family & Society Studies Worldwide <http://www.nisc.com>* 1997
- *Family Index Database <http://www.familyscholar.com>* 2004
- *Health & Psychosocial Instruments (HaPI) Database (available through online and as a CD-ROM from Ovid Technologies)* .... *
- *Index Guide to College Journals (core list compiled by integrating 48 indexes frequently used to support undergraduate programs in small to medium-sized libraries)* 1999
- *Occupational Therapy Database (OTDBASE) has a user friendly index created so that each abstract can be found easily & quickly. Subscriptions can be obtained at www.otdbase.com <http://www.otdbase.com>* 1980
- *Occupational Therapy Index/AMED Database* 1993
- *OCLC ArticleFirst <http://www.oclc.org/services/databases/>* 2002
- *OCLC ContentsFirst <http://www.oclc.org/services/databases/>* ... 2002
- *OTseeker <http://www.otseeker.com>* 2002
- *OT SEARCH <http://www.aota.org/otsearch/>* 1991
- *Psychiatric Rehabilitation Journal* 1997
- *Social Work Abstracts <http://www.silverplatter.com/catalog/swab.htm>* 1982
- *SocIndex (EBSCO)* 2003
- *Sociological Abstracts (SA) <http://www.csa.com>* .... *
- *SPORTDiscus <http://www.sportquest.com/>* 1994
- *SwetsNet <http://www.swetsnet.com>* 2001

* **Exact start date to come.**

(continued)

Special Bibliographic Notes related to special journal issues
(separates) and indexing/abstracting:

- indexing/abstracting services in this list will also cover material in any "separate" that is co-published simultaneously with Haworth's special thematic journal issue or DocuSerial. Indexing/abstracting usually covers material at the article/chapter level.
- monographic co-editions are intended for either non-subscribers or libraries which intend to purchase a second copy for their circulating collections.
- monographic co-editions are reported to all jobbers/wholesalers/approval plans. The source journal is listed as the "series" to assist the prevention of duplicate purchasing in the same manner utilized for books-in-series.
- to facilitate user/access services all indexing/abstracting services are encouraged to utilize the co-indexing entry note indicated at the bottom of the first page of each article/chapter/contribution.
- this is intended to assist a library user of any reference tool (whether print, electronic, online, or CD-ROM) to locate the monographic version if the library has purchased this version but not a subscription to the source journal.
- individual articles/chapters in any Haworth publication are also available through the Haworth Document Delivery Service (HDDS).

Occupational Therapy in Forensic Psychiatry: Role Development and Schizophrenia

CONTENTS

Preface   XV

Chapter 1. Introduction: Social Roles and Schizophrenia
    in Forensic Psychiatry   1

Chapter 2. Typical Development of Roles and the Impact
    of Schizophrenia on the Development of Adult Social Roles   11

Chapter 3. Role Development: Treatment Guidelines   25

Chapter 4. Implementing Role Development:
    Tools and Resources   47

Chapter 5. Designing an Outcomes-Based Research Study
    to Assess the Development of Roles in Adults Diagnosed
    with Schizophrenia   57

Chapter 6. Evaluating the Effectiveness of Role Development:
    Quantitative Data   79

Chapter 7. Evaluating the Effectiveness
    of Role Development: Qualitative Data   105

Chapter 8. Case Studies   111

Chapter 9. Response of the Rehabilitation Staff
   to Role Development   123

Chapter 10. An Analysis of the Effectiveness
   of the Intervention   133

References   151

APPENDICES

Appendix A   163

Appendix B   165

Index   177

ABOUT THE AUTHOR

Victoria P. Schindler, PhD, OTR, is Assistant Professor of Occupational Therapy at the Richard Stockton College of New Jersey. Dr. Schindler has worked in the area of mental health occupational therapy for over 20 years in settings including inpatient and outpatient psychiatric facilities and a maximum security forensic facility. Dr. Schindler has a BS in occupational therapy (Kean University), a post-professional MA in occupational therapy (New York University) and a PhD in occupational therapy (New York University).

ACKNOWLEDGMENTS

I would like to thank Deborah Labovitz, PhD, OTR, Judy Grossman, PhD, OTR, Mary Donohue, PhD, OTR and the faculty at New York University for their guidance and support. I would also like to thank the staff at the facility in which the study took place for their willingness to participate in implementing the intervention and in data collection. Lastly, I would like to thank the patients who so generously participated in the study. They were an inspiration to me. This book was derived from research completed for my doctoral degree at New York University.

Preface

This volume, *Occupational Therapy in Forensic Psychiatry: Role Development and Schizophrenia*, includes a description of a set of guidelines for clinical practice, Role Development, a research study that assessed the effectiveness of this set of guidelines, and practical information and resources for therapists to implement this set of guidelines with their clients.

Role Development is based on the concept of social roles. Social roles are the foundation of all social behaviors. Individuals learn social roles, such as worker, family member, and friend, throughout their lives, and roles can be learned in a functional or dysfunctional manner (Parsons, 1951). Effective role functioning requires a repertoire of task and interpersonal skills.

The learning of effective roles and skills can be disrupted in individuals diagnosed with a schizophrenic disorder. Commonly available treatment, such as medication and activity programs, may alleviate symptoms and promote improvement for these individuals, but may not address the development of social roles or skills. Additional treatment methods are required to develop roles and skills (Lehman & Steinwachs, 1998). One such method is treatment based on a set of guidelines for clinical practice (Mosey, 1996).

Role Development (Schindler, 2002), a set of guidelines for clinical practice, provides direction for health care practitioners to assist individuals diagnosed with schizophrenic disorders to learn social roles and the task and interpersonal skills associated with these roles.

[Haworth co-indexing entry note]: "Preface." Schindler, Victoria P. Co-published simultaneously in *Occupational Therapy in Mental Health* (The Haworth Press, Inc.) Vol. 20, No. 3/4, 2004, pp. xvii-xviii and: *Occupational Therapy in Forensic Psychiatry: Role Development and Schizophrenia* (Victoria P. Schindler) The Haworth Press, Inc., 2004, pp. xv-xvi. Single or multiple copies of this article are available for a fee from The Haworth Document Delivery Service [1-800-HAWORTH, 9:00 a.m. - 5:00 p.m. (EST). E-mail address: docdelivery@haworthpress.com].

The research problem in this study was to ascertain if individuals diagnosed with schizophrenic disorders demonstrated greater improvement in task and interpersonal skills and social roles when involved in the Role Development program in comparison to a multi-departmental activity program. A pretest-posttest design with repeated measures follow-up at four, eight, and 12 weeks was used. Three rating scales and one self-perception checklist were used as data collection instruments. Participants were 84 adult males, diagnosed with a schizophrenic disorder, and confined to a maximum-security psychiatric facility. Eighteen rehabilitation staff members were trained in Role Development, and they provided this intervention to participants in the experimental group.

Data analysis included quantitative and qualitative results. There were no demographic differences between participants in the experimental and comparison groups. Within-group tests, between-group tests, ANCOVA, MANCOVA, and repeated measures ANOVA were conducted. Data analysis indicated that participants in the Role Development program showed statistically significant improvement in the development of task skills, interpersonal skills, and role functioning, especially at four weeks of treatment, in comparison to participants in the multi-departmental activity program. Qualitative data from staff focus groups and patient interviews supported the findings.

Case studies are provided to demonstrate application of Role Development to individuals diagnosed with schizophrenia. Finally, a description of Role Development and forms to facilitate the practical use of this set of guidelines have been included.

Chapter 1

Introduction:
Social Roles and Schizophrenia
in Forensic Psychiatry

INTRODUCTION

Paul is a single, 20-year-old male, of Italian and African American descent. He was incarcerated following an altercation with his father and at the jail appeared to be responding to internal stimuli. Paul had resided with his parents and younger brother and sister ages 19 and 15 respectively. Both parents worked at a factory.

Paul completed the 11th grade at a Technical Institute and was a few months into 12th grade when he started to become withdrawn, isolative and paranoid. He refused to attend school and became more reclusive at home. In a short time he quit school and did not earn a high school diploma or a GED. He had one job as a busboy at a chain restaurant, but he quickly became suspicious of others and was absent from work. After only a few weeks he was fired for absenteeism. He began to argue with his parents more as their frustration with him grew.

Paul's family denied any history of alcohol or substance abuse or mental illness or legal problems. Paul denied any history of physical or sexual abuse. Paul also denied any history of substance abuse. He stated

---

[Haworth co-indexing entry note]: "Introduction: Social Roles and Schizophrenia in Forensic Psychiatry." Schindler, Victoria P. Co-published simultaneously in *Occupational Therapy in Mental Health* (The Haworth Press, Inc.) Vol. 20, No. 3/4, 2004, pp. 1-9; and: *Occupational Therapy in Forensic Psychiatry: Role Development and Schizophrenia* (Victoria P. Schindler) The Haworth Press, Inc., 2004, pp. 1-9. Single or multiple copies of this article are available for a fee from The Haworth Document Delivery Service [1-800-HAWORTH, 9:00 a.m. - 5:00 p.m. (EST). E-mail address: docdelivery@haworthpress.com].

that he had tried alcohol but denied using it on a regular basis. He denied blackouts and denied using marijuana, cocaine, heroin, or other drugs. Records suggest that he might have used marijuana in the past but he denied such use. He had never been referred to, or treated in, a drug rehabilitation facility.

Paul had difficulty believing that he may have symptoms of schizophrenia. He repeatedly stated his belief that he does not need to take medications. He reported that the medication has no impact on him, stating, "I feel the same with medication as without medication." In addition to the growing problems Paul was experiencing at home, Paul also stated he didn't have any friends or anyone with whom he could confide or talk.

Paul reported that his current legal problems resulted from an "argument" with his father. He stated that he was lying on the couch with his eyes closed, and his father was talking to him about getting a job and not lying around the house. Reportedly, his father threw a book at him, and "I started yelling at him." His mother and brother apparently tried to break up the fight. The police were called, arrested Paul, and charged him with harassment. Records indicate that such altercations have occurred in the past.

Paul's family and the police subsequently dropped all charges. However, Paul's family did not want him to return home. They stated he could only return home when he was settled in a job.

Young men who are Paul's age typically have several coexisting roles such as student, worker, friend, son, brother, and boyfriend, significant other or spouse. However, Paul had none of these roles. He had quit high school and did not have a GED, was unsuccessful at the only short-term job he had held, had no friends nor a significant other, and was becoming increasingly distanced and uncomfortable as a family member. In fact, an argument with his father resulted in Paul's arrest and commitment to a forensic hospital. For a young man who would typically have several roles indicating a developing, fulfilling life, Paul's current roles were limited to patient and inmate. The symptoms of schizophrenia not only invaded Paul with frightening, paranoid, and unreal thoughts, but also robbed him of his ability to function normally in roles typical of young men his age.

Roles are patterns of behavior and the foundation of all social behavior (Parsons, 1951a), and they are commonly referred to as social roles (Barbour & Moreno, 1980; Blume, Green, Joanning, & Quinn, 1994; Karmel, 1970; Ruddock, 1976; Wapner & Craig-Bray, 1992). Social roles have also been defined as a combination of behaviors, functions, privileges, and responsibilities that are socially defined and expected of an individual in a particular position in society (Wolfensberger, 2000). Social roles are not roles one plays in the theater or personality roles, such as that of a leader or a follower, but life roles that are the foundation of our relationships with our families, friends, work, and community. Some social roles are spouse, community member, student, and friend (Kielhofner, 1985, 1995; Mosey, 1986). Such roles are potent because we attach considerable importance to them (Anthony & Liberman, 1986; Durkheim, 1938; Pearlin, 1983). These roles are also basic to all interactions and relate to all areas of human experience including family life, activities of daily living, school/work, and play/leisure/recreation (Kielhofner, 1995; Mosey, 1986). Enacting roles that are important and meaningful to us produces contentment, joy, and satisfaction (Csikszentmihalyi & Csikszentmihalyi, 1988; Mead, 1964; Sarbin & Scheibe, 1983).

Individuals learn social roles throughout their lives in a developmental manner and normally act out a number of different roles at the same time. These roles can vary in priority at different times in the life cycle (Ruddock, 1976; Sarbin & Scheibe, 1983). For example, a 35-year-old man may have active roles of a husband, father, son, brother, worker, and basketball coach for his daughter's team. The role of basketball coach may be dropped if his daughter loses interest in the game. Although the thought of juggling simultaneous roles may spark overwhelming feelings of frustration, individuals with a variety of roles in their repertoire are often better able to function in society because they can deal with a wide range of situations (Stephan & Stephan, 1990; Thoits, 1983).

Roles can be learned in a functional or dysfunctional manner. An individual can be highly adept at performing many aspects of a role or can be lacking in skills or motivation to perform a role successfully and consistently. For example, the role of parent can be developed in a way that is supportive and nurturing to a child or in a way that is harmful or neglectful. Roles are generally beneficial to society. However, an individual can also learn a role that is considered deviant, such as that of a criminal (Karmel, 1970; Parsons, 1951a; Wolfensberger, 2000).

To enact a role effectively, individuals need a repertoire of task and interpersonal skills, and these skills are the foundation of roles (Black, 1976; Liberman et al., 1993; Mosey, 1986; Versluys, 1980). Task skills that are basic to roles include paying attention, following directions, and solving problems related to a task. Interpersonal skills include initiating and sustaining a conversation and expressing one's thoughts and feelings. For example, a restaurant cook needs to be able to follow directions for various recipes, interact with peers, and relate to supervisors appropriately. When task and interpersonal skills are learned in a functional manner, learning is hierarchical, and the learning of basic skills precedes the learning of complex skills. For example, one must be willing to engage in a task prior to being able to follow the directions associated with that task. However, just like social roles, task and interpersonal skills can be learned in a dysfunctional manner, or not at all (Mosey, 1986).

The development of roles can be disrupted in individuals diagnosed with a mental illness. The more disabling the mental illness, the more it affects the learning of and ability to sustain social roles (Anthony, 1993; Parsons, 1951b; Pearlin, 1983; Shannon, 1972; Wessen, 1965; Wolfensberger, 2000). One of the most severe types of mental illness is the schizophrenic disorders. Schizophrenic disorders are classified as a group of psychotic disorders that cause a major disturbance of personality. This disturbance takes the form of positive symptoms (i.e., primary symptoms), such as delusions and hallucinations, and negative symptoms (i.e., secondary symptoms), such as apathy, withdrawal, and avolition (American Psychiatric Association, *Diagnostic and Statistical Manual of Mental Disorders-IV [DSM-IV]*, 1994; Straube & Oades, 1992; World Health Organization [WHO], 1978).

Schizophrenia involves dysfunction in one or more major areas such as interpersonal relations, work or education, or self-care (*DSM-IV*, 1994, p. 277). The overwhelming effects of the sequelae of schizophrenia can clearly affect an individual's ability to learn or carry out social roles. Individuals diagnosed with schizophrenic disorders are often limited by their symptoms in their ability to function as a parent, lover, shopper, or friend, or engage in other roles that would be meaningful to someone of their age or gender. Social roles are either never developed or are withdrawn or severed. Wolfensberger (2000) describes individuals with severe mental illness as persons who often do not have a single positive role involving an enduring unpaid relationship.

To complicate matters further, some of the few remaining roles enacted by individuals diagnosed with schizophrenic disorders are viewed as dysfunctional by society. One of these roles is that of patient. This role can be viewed as dysfunctional because it involves a pattern of passive, dependent behavior as opposed to active, independent behavior (Parsons, 1951b; Pearlin, 1983; Wessen, 1965; Wolfensberger, 2000). In addition, individuals diagnosed with schizophrenic disorders often have deficits in learning and/or maintaining the task and interpersonal skills necessary to enact positive, socially acceptable roles. These basic skill deficits are manifested in areas such as personal hygiene, money management, eating habits, cooking skills, use of public transportation, and use of leisure time (Broekema, Danz, & Schloemer, 1975; Liberman et al., 1993; Mann et al., 1993).

For individuals diagnosed with schizophrenic disorders, commonly available treatment such as medication and activity programs may alleviate symptoms and promote involvement in activity and social interactions. However, activity programs may not address the development of social roles or the specific skills that are nested in these roles. Additional treatment methods are required to develop these skills and roles (Lehman & Steinwachs, 1998). One such method is treatment based on a set of guidelines for clinical practice. Sets of guidelines for practice describe the assessment and intervention methods necessary to promote change within a specific theoretical foundation. Staff trained in the use of a set of guidelines for practice are then able to use their skills and knowledge to facilitate positive growth and change in their clients (Mosey, 1996).

Role Development (see Chapter 3) (Schindler, 2002), a set of guidelines for clinical practice, has been developed to provide direction for health care practitioners in assisting individuals diagnosed with schizophrenic disorders to learn social roles and their underlying task and interpersonal skills. As with all sets of guidelines for practice, Role Development links theory to practice and consists of four parts: theoretical base, function-dysfunction continuums, behaviors indicative of function and dysfunction, and methods to promote positive change. The theoretical base of Role Development focuses on an individual's need to learn and feel competent and successful in social roles. It describes how learning takes place, the learning of typical and atypical roles, and the therapeutic tools that assist in the process of learning roles. The continuums and the behaviors indicative of function and dysfunction address skills (task and interpersonal) and roles (worker, student, group member, friend). The postulates to promote positive change are the specific ways to design the intervention to engage the client in the development of roles (Kielhofner, 1985, 1995; Mosey, 1986, 1996).

The primary source for Role Development is Role Acquisition, a frame of reference developed by Mosey (1986). Role Acquisition was developed in 1986 and used with individuals diagnosed with psychiatric illnesses–particularly with individuals residing in the community or anticipating a return to the community in the near future (Mosey, 1986, p. 450).

In contrast, this study was implemented in a maximum-security psychiatric facility. Individuals hospitalized in this type of facility often have fewer and less independent roles than others of their age and gender (Parsons, 1951b; Pearlin, 1983; Sarbin & Scheibe, 1983; Wessen, 1965). Some of these individuals have been hospitalized or incarcerated for much of their adult lives, whereas others have lived in community environments plagued with abuse, neglect, alcohol, and illicit drugs. As a result, many of these individuals have not developed constructive social roles; others have developed social roles but no longer perform them. The development of roles needs to begin at a level lower than that described in Role Acquisition. Therefore, to better meet the needs of the patients in this study, the Role Acquisition frame of reference was modified, resulting in Role Development.

Role Acquisition was modified in several ways. The theoretical base of Role Acquisition consisted primarily of Mosey's original work. This was expanded upon in Role Development to include some of the seminal literature on role theory (Durkheim, 1938; Mead, 1964; Merton, 1957; Parsons, 1951a; Sarbin, 1954), social learning theory (Bandura, 1977), and skill development (Anthony, 1993; Fidler, 1969; Liberman et al., 1993). Additionally, the function-dysfunction continuums in Role Acquisition addressed task and interpersonal skills on an equal level with roles and included the areas of activities of daily living, play/leisure/recreation, and family interaction. In Role Development, task and interpersonal skills are nested within roles. In the maximum-security psychiatric facility in which this study was implemented, patients are not allowed access to some of the types of settings associated with activities of daily living, play/leisure/recreation, and family interaction (e.g., one's own home, community recreational facilities). Therefore, Role Development does not address activities of daily living or family interaction, and has incorporated some of the aspects of play/leisure/recreation into the role of friend. Also, Role Development has included the role of group member.

For the individuals involved in this study, the road to developing constructive social roles, and the tasks and interpersonal skills nested within these roles, may be a long one. First, in institutions such as the one in this study, the number and type of roles one can develop is restricted (Sarbin & Scheibe, 1983). This study addressed roles that are attainable in this setting such as student, worker, friend, and group member. Also, because the roles of individuals in this setting may have been severely limited in the past, learning of roles, and the skills associated with these roles, may be slower and take longer to develop. Lastly, for a variety of legal reasons, individuals hospitalized in a maximum-security setting have varying lengths of stay. Some individuals may stay in the setting for only a few weeks, whereas others may stay for several years. Usually, less can be practiced and learned in weeks than in years. Although this must be considered, it is important that the learning process is initiated. Therapeutic interventions should not be ignored or excused due to short-term hospitalizations or more complex needs of the individuals requiring services (Stuve & Menditto, 1999). With these factors in mind, the following problem statement and hypotheses were developed.

PROBLEM STATEMENT

The rationale for this study is that health care practitioners need to provide meaningful, relevant interventions, and empirical information regarding the effectiveness of these interventions, to clients receiving health care services and the payers of these services. The purpose of this study was to examine the effectiveness of an intervention, Role Development, on the development of task and interpersonal skills and social roles in adults diagnosed with schizophrenic disorders. Because there is no empirical information on this set of guidelines for practice, this study was the first step in examining the effectiveness of Role Development as a frame of reference or guideline for practice.

HYPOTHESES Archive Friday it no Hand. 0

Adults diagnosed with schizophrenic disorders demonstrate greater improvement in task skills (as evidenced by a statistically significant improvement in scores on the Task Skills Scale) when involved in an individualized intervention based on Role Development in comparison to participation in a multidepartmental activity program.

Adults diagnosed with schizophrenic disorders demonstrate greater improvement in interpersonal skills (as evidenced by a statistically significant improvement in scores on the Interpersonal Skills Scale) when involved in an individualized intervention based on Role Development in comparison to participation in a multidepartmental activity program.

Adults diagnosed with schizophrenic disorders develop more social roles (as evidenced by a statistically significant improvement in scores on the Role Functioning Scale and a greater number of roles on the Role Checklist) when involved in an individualized intervention based on Role Development in comparison to participation in a multidepartmental activity program.

The longer an individual participates in treatment based on Role Development, the greater will be the difference between his scores on the three scales (Task Skills Scale, Interpersonal Skills Scale and Role Functioning Scale) and those of persons participating in a multidepartmental activity program.

DEFINITIONS

Role Development Program is an intervention based on a theoretical set of guidelines for practice that addresses the development of meaningful social roles and the skills that are the foundation of these roles. It is an individualized intervention in which staff and client work collaboratively to identify and develop the client's social roles, such as worker, student, friend, and group member, and the task and interpersonal skills associated with these roles. When the Role Development Program is implemented by a variety of rehabilitation staff members, it provides a common link and theoretical foundation on which to base intervention (Kielhofner, 1985; Mosey, 1986; Schindler, 2002). Role Development Program is defined operationally as the set of guidelines for practice used to address the development of social roles and the task and interpersonal skills associated with these roles (see Chapter 3).

Social Roles are life roles that are the foundation of our relationships with our families, work, and community, such as worker, group member, student, and friend (Mosey, 1986; Wolfensberger, 2000). Social roles are defined operationally as the score an individual receives on the adapted Role Functioning Scale (Goodman, Sewell, Cooley, & Leavitt, 1993) and the roles an individual chooses to address on the adapted Role Checklist (Oakley, 1981).

Task Skills are physical and cognitive abilities used to manipulate the nonhuman environment (Mosey, 1986, p. 451). Task skills are defined operationally as the score an individual receives on the Task Skills Scale (Mosey, 1986, pp. 322 & 453) during the performance of structured activities.

Interpersonal Skills are verbal and non-verbal abilities used to interact in dyadic and group situations. Interpersonal skills are defined operationally as the score an individual receives on the Interpersonal Skills Scale (Mosey, 1986, pp. 324 & 454; Rogers, Sciarappa, & Anthony, 1991) during interaction with others in the course of structured activities.

The Comparison Group consists of two subgroups: *Multi-departmental Activity Program* is a non-individualized, therapeutic intervention designed to encourage the productive use of time and socialization in a group setting. Individuals in this program are scheduled to participate in leisure, education, and work-oriented activity groups. Intervention is group-oriented and is *not* structured to address the development of individual social roles or the specific skills that are nested in these roles. There is no common link or theoretical foundation among staff using this intervention. The Multidepartmental Activity Program is the routine activity-based program implemented in this facility prior to this study. *Multi-departmental Activity Program* is defined operationally as the four one-hour programs comprising a patient's daily program schedule in the maximum-security facility in which this study occurred (Clark et al., 1997).

Multi-departmental Activity Program with Individual Attention is the same activity program described above with the addition of a weekly 15-minute individual social session between staff and the individual. The purpose of this social session is to give individual attention to the patient in the form of social conversation. Individuals in this program are also scheduled to participate in leisure, education, and work-oriented activity groups. Multi-departmental Activity Program with Individual Attention is defined operationally as the four one-hour programs comprising a patient's daily program schedule with the weekly 15-minute social session in the maximum-security facility in which this study will occur (Clark et al., 1997).

Schizophrenic Disorders are a group of disorders characterized by positive symptoms (i.e., primary symptoms) such as delusions, hallucinations, disorganized speech and grossly disorganized or catatonic behavior, and negative symptoms (i.e., secondary symptoms) such as affective flattening, avolition, and alogia, causing a deterioration in social and occupational functioning for a duration of at least six months (*DSM-IV-R*, 2000; Straube & Oades, 1992; World Health Organization [WHO], 1978). Schizophrenic Disorders are defined operationally as those disorders listed in the DSM-IV Axis I diagnosis of the client's hospital record as Schizophrenia, undifferentiated type; Schizophrenia, residual type; Schizophrenia, catatonic type; Schizophrenia, paranoid type; and Schizoaffective disorder.

Statistically Significant. For clarification, the use of the term "statistically significant" throughout this journal defines a statistically significant result at $p < .05$.

Chapter 2

Typical Development of Roles and the Impact of Schizophrenia on the Development of Adult Social Roles

The development of roles is a universal process that continues through the course of our lives. Typical development of roles has been discussed by many theorists and related to significant events (e.g., marriage) and to the stages (e.g., adulthood) of our lives. Much has also been written about the manner in which typical development of roles can be adversely affected by trauma, injury, and illness, such as schizophrenia. This chapter will explore typical and atypical development of roles by addressing four areas: role theory, the development of roles in individuals diagnosed with schizophrenic disorders, the development of task and interpersonal skills in relation to the development of roles in forensic settings, and the development and documented use of Role Development.

ROLE THEORY

An historical review of role theory begins in the 1930s and continues to evolve today. The concept of role originated in drama in the form of a wooden scroll on which the actor's lines were written. This concept was

[Haworth co-indexing entry note]: "Typical Development of Roles and the Impact of Schizophrenia on the Development of Adult Social Roles." Schindler, Victoria P. Co-published simultaneously in *Occupational Therapy in Mental Health* (The Haworth Press, Inc.) Vol. 20, No. 3/4, 2004, pp. 11-23; and: *Occupational Therapy in Forensic Psychiatry: Role Development and Schizophrenia* (Victoria P. Schindler) The Haworth Press, Inc., 2004, pp. 11-23. Single or multiple copies of this article are available for a fee from The Haworth Document Delivery Service [1-800-HAWORTH, 9:00 a.m. - 5:00 p.m. (EST). E-mail address: docdelivery@haworthpress.com].

http://www.haworthpress.com/web/OTMH
Digital Object Identifier: 10.1300/J004v20n03_02

adopted by social psychologists and applied to role theory (Landy, 1991). Information on the development and use of role theory dates to the 1930s and demonstrates changes in the conceptual understanding of the theory as it progresses to the current time.

The evolution of role theory focused on two schools of thought: structural functionalism and symbolic interactionism. Both approaches borrowed language from the theater and used the term "role" to describe the parts individuals play as they live their lives (Schumacher, 1995). Linton (1936) was one of the early writers of role theory and one of the first contributors to structural functionalism. He viewed roles as the expected behaviors of an individual's status or position in a social structure. Other structural functionalists (Durkheim, 1938; Merton, 1957; Parsons, 1951) expanded this theory around a central concept of scripts. Scripts are norms for behavior and are inherent to any position within a society. Behavior is determined by the surrounding social structure. Structural functionalism operates at the macroscopic level; it is evidenced through the norms, values, structure, and cultural rules of a society (deMarrias & LeCompte, 1995). Two decades later Sarbin (1954) further expanded this theory by defining roles as patterns of behaviors that are learned through intentional instruction and incidental learning. This learning of roles begins in a child as play. Reinforcement or a reward/punishment system accompanies this type of learning. As the child grows, he/she develops a set of expectations regarding roles.

Symbolic interactionism, to the contrary, views scripts as providing only a broad guide for action. This theory proposes that human behavior is attributable more to an individual's unique characteristics and perceptions than to an overlying social structure. Proponents of symbolic interactionism state that behavior is based on evolving interactions between actors. Roles are associated with identities rather than social positions. In this theory, individuals, rather than society, are active in shaping their environments and futures. Symbolic interactionism functions at the microscopic level; it is evidenced through the continual, everyday realities of social interactions (Blumer, 1969; deMarrias & LeCompte, 1995; Mead, 1964).

Structural functionalism and symbolic interactionism continued to influence role theory for several decades. In the 1970s, information on role theory expanded to address specific roles and the complexity of role theory. Heise and Roberts (1970) continued the development of role knowledge by describing a variety of family and occupational roles and by developing an instrument to measure role knowledge. The authors developed a tool that paired 15 role names with 20 behaviors.

They administered this tool to both children and adults, and concluded that age, sibling structure, contact and exposure, and authoritarianism are more integral to role learning than sex and intelligence. The authors also concluded that at least two-thirds of measured adult role knowledge is acquired by seven years of age.

Ruddock (1976) introduced the concept of variance within roles. Although there may be certain expectations associated with a role, he believed that individuals vary in the way they enact their roles. Depending on one's degree of comfort, motivation, and satisfaction with a role, an individual may show varying degrees of identification with, or distance from, a role. Although some of these concepts were introduced at earlier times, other authors (Biddle, 1979; Grace, 1972; Gross, Mason, & McEachern, 1958; Hardy & Conway, 1978; Levin, 1994; Pearlin, 1983) further developed and expanded concepts such as role set (a set of roles performed by a person), role overload (a set of roles that is too complex), role conflict (discrepancies in the expectations within one role or between two or more roles), role strain (stress associated with the expectations of a role), and role incongruity (expectations for role performance that are counter to attitudes, disposition, or values).

Social learning theory (Bandura, 1977) also had an impact on the development of role theory. Central concepts such as modeling, reinforcement, punishment, and consequences, can be applied to the way in which one learns a role. In learning roles, children model behavior of older children or adults, receive positive or negative reinforcement for their behavior, and subsequently alter or continue their behavior. In one study, Bandura (1977, p. 120) found that children who saw assaultive behavior consistently rewarded became aggressive as they grew older. Unfortunately, aggressive behavior can later be incorporated in the role of parent, worker, or friend.

Another type of development in the area of role theory was the focus on roles within groups or group membership roles (Parsons & Bales, 1955). The development of theory on these group roles began in 1955 and continued through the 1970s. These group membership roles took the form of group task roles and group social-emotional roles. Examples of group task roles are initiator-contributor, information seeker, and coordinator. Examples of social-emotional roles are encourager, compromiser, gatekeeper, and follower. These are roles an individual plays in a group. Some of these roles will provide a positive contribution to a group while other roles can impede the progress of a group. For example, an individual who wants to be the center of attention of the group can slow the flow of group process. Although this work on roles does not directly contribute to the literature on social roles, it did make an important contribution to the literature on role theory (Benne & Sheats, 1978; Howe & Schwartzberg, 1995; Mosey, 1973).

Minimal theoretical information and no empirical studies were found on role theory during the 1980s. In fact, one author reported that with a few exceptions, role theory was dormant during the past three decades and direct tests of role theory, at any time, are rare (George, 1993). Some authors believe that the diminished popularity of role theory is due to its lack of clear connection between theory and practice (George, 1993; Kipper, 1991). However, in 1985, Stryker and Statham proposed an integrated model of role theory. Instead of viewing structural functionalism and symbolic interactionism as incompatible, the authors viewed the two theories as complementary. They proposed that individuals blend social expectations with creative, unique approaches to develop roles.

Stronger interest in role theory appears to have resumed in the 1990s until today. Role theory has become more complex and more directly relevant to life situations and transitions (Callero, 1994; George, 1993; Kipper, 1991; Wapner & Craig-Bray, 1992). For example, whereas in the past it was widely held that multiple roles promoted negative reactions such as role strain or role conflict, current thinking is that a variety of roles can have a positive influence on an individual's ability to function in society. Multiple roles equip a person to deal with a wide variety of situations and to compensate for disappointment in one role by succeeding in other roles (Stephan & Stephan, 1990). Thoits (1993) found that individuals who hold numerous social roles reported less psychological distress than those holding few roles. Resources, such as social contacts in one role, were used to meet obligations of other roles. During the adult stage (age 30-50) when individuals normally hold the most roles, a variety of roles are important. In another effort to reinvigorate role theory, Callero (1994) viewed roles as a vehicle to expand one's options rather than a consequence of one's position (e.g., the role of college professor is used to achieve membership on editorial boards). Recently, Wolfensberger (2000) developed Social Role Valorization, a theory that addresses individuals who are considered to be devalued by their society such as the mentally ill, the poor, and prisoners. This theory describes the plight of persons considered devalued and offers some broad recommendations to change this societal view and improve life conditions of persons in these circumstances.

Role theory has evolved over the past 60 years. Originating from two schools of thought (structural functionalism and symbolic interactionism), role theory has gained depth as it has added concepts reflecting the current complexities of role functioning. Role theory currently describes multiple roles, a variety of facets of individual roles, and conveys the centrality of roles in an individual's life.

THE DEVELOPMENT OF ROLES IN INDIVIDUALS DIAGNOSED WITH SCHIZOPHRENIC DISORDERS

Typically, the learning of roles follows a developmental progression. This begins in childhood, the number and intensity of roles peaks between age 30-60, and then the number of roles declines as one gets closer to death (Black, 1976; Matsutsuyu, 1971; Thoits, 1983). This normal development of roles can be severely hindered by mental illness.

Schizophrenia can be a devastating mental illness. It affects about 1% of the population and more than 75% of individuals diagnosed with schizophrenia will experience mental impairments throughout their life. About two million people currently living in the United States will be affected by schizophrenia during their lifetime. Although schizophrenia affects women and men equally, its onset usually occurs between ages 20 and 30 for men and somewhat later for women (Straube & Oades, 1992; World Health Organization [WHO], 1978). This is typically a time in one's life for developing multiple roles (Black, 1976; Matsutsuyu, 1971; Thoits, 1983).

Schizophrenic disorders have positive symptoms (i.e., primary symptoms), such as delusions and hallucinations, and negative symptoms (i.e., secondary symptoms), such as apathy, withdrawal, and avolition. The positive symptoms must persist for one month or longer to warrant the diagnosis of schizophrenia (*DSM-IV-R*, 2000; Straube & Oades, 1992; WHO, 1978).

Delusions manifest as characteristic distortions of thinking that present as bizarre, erroneous beliefs. A greatly disturbing but common delusion is a belief that, despite the absence of surgical scars, one's internal body parts or organs, such as the brain or uterus, were removed and replaced with one of an animal or another person. Delusions usually focus on themes. Common themes are of a persecutory or referential nature (*DSM-IV-R*, 2000; Straube & Oades, 1992).

Hallucinations present as a sensory disturbance in any of the sensory functions (i.e., auditory, visual, olfactory, gustatory, and tactile), but auditory hallucinations are the most common. Auditory hallucinations are perceived as voices within one's brain that are different from one's own thoughts or conscience. Voices can be from a person who is familiar or unfamiliar to the individual, or two or more voices can occur simultaneously or converse with each other. Although some voices can be innocuous, individuals experiencing voices usually describe them as disparaging or outright threatening (*DSM-IV-R,* 2000; Straube & Oades, 1992).

Other positive symptoms of schizophrenia include disorganized thinking, grossly disorganized behavior, and catatonic motor behaviors. Disorganized thinking may present as an inability to stay focused on a topic to the point that an individual is skipping from one topic to another so that the conversation no longer makes any sense, or the individual may use sounds, words or phrases that are incomprehensible. Grossly disorganized behavior can range from silliness to unpredictable agitation. It may also manifest as very poor hygiene, bizarre or inappropriate dress (e.g., multiple layers of clothes on a hot day), or outbursts of loud or agitated behavior. Catatonic motor behaviors manifest as bizarre postures, excessive, repetitive motor activity or extremely slow motor responses to stimuli in the environment (*DSM-IV-R,* 2000).

The negative symptoms of schizophrenia can be equally disabling. The three most common negative symptoms are affective flattening, alogia, and avolition. The face of an individual experiencing affective flattening will appear immobile and unresponsive, and his or her range of emotional expressiveness will be clearly diminished. Alogia is also known as poverty of speech and is manifested by brief, empty replies and an overall decrease in the productivity of speech. Avolition is an inability to initiate or maintain goal-directed activity (*DSM-IV-R,* 2000). An individual demonstrating this symptom may lie in bed for hours, day after day, with no interest in task or social activities.

Symptoms of schizophrenia can have a severe impact on an individual's ability to learn social roles. A number of researchers recognized the difference between functional and dysfunctional roles and the impact of chronic disability on role acquisition (Anthony, 1993; Anthony & Liberman, 1986; Gove & Lubach, 1968; Heard, 1977; Karmel, 1970; Susser, Stein, Mountey, & Freeman, 1970).

Sick Role

Parsons (1951b) introduced the "sick" role, and Ludwig and Adams (1968) examined factors that led to appropriate use or misuse of this role. In addressing the psychiatric population, several authors found that once individuals with psychiatric illnesses are removed from their community environments and are institutionalized for long periods of time, they lose many of their social roles and cannot reenter the community and start where they left off. Instead, many of these individuals learn roles that are deviant or passive in nature and do not promote independent functioning in the community (Dickerson & Oakley, 1985; Goffman, 1961; Gove & Lubach, 1968; Heard, 1977; Karmel, 1970; Pearlin, 1983; Shannon, 1972; Susser, Stein, Mountey, & Freeman, 1970; Versluys, 1980; Wolfensberger, 2000). During the 1960s when hospitalizations averaged four to six months, Gove and Lubach (1968) developed and tested a pilot program to counter the traditional long-term stay for individuals with psychiatric illnesses including schizophrenia. This pilot program had a set of distinct treatment stages, including a system whereby each patient received high intramuscular dosages of medication within an hour of admission, all patients kept and used personal belongings, wards were gender-mixed, and a close involvement of family was initiated upon admission. The pilot program assessed the participants' roles upon their return to the community. In comparing the pilot group of 258 patients to a historical control group of 171 patients, the authors found that the individuals in the pilot group had a length of stay that was one-half that of the control group, were better able to retain their family roles during the year following admission, and were more likely to return to a worker role upon their return to the community.

Other researchers addressed the interference of hospitalization and the consequent separation from one's family and community roles on an individual's ability to develop meaningful roles. One group of researchers (Sood, Baker, & Bledin, 1996) compared the skills and roles of inpatients with stays between six months and five years (new long-stay patients) with discharged patients who had resided in the community for a similar length of time (new long-term patients). Schizophrenia was the primary diagnosis for both groups. Both groups were found to have similar deficits in skills and roles pertaining to the community and social relations, but the new long-stay patients were found to have more deficits in self-care and domestic skills.

Social Network Therapy

A few authors assessed areas of functioning related to roles in individuals diagnosed with schizophrenia. In recognizing a connection between social networks and satisfying social roles, 25 individuals diagnosed with schizophrenia were examined after one year of social network therapy (i.e., structured therapy process to assist individuals in expanding and enhancing their social relationships); 12 showed improvement in their social network with an increase in the number of reciprocal relationships and confidants (Gillies et al., 1993). Another group of researchers developed a psycho-educational program aimed at decreasing the severity of illness and improving community functioning and quality of life. Although roles were not directly assessed, satisfaction with roles was linked to successful community functioning and positive quality of life. The majority of participants in this preliminary study demonstrated reduced psychopathology and improved community functioning (Halford et al., 1995). Other authors (Brekke, Long, Nesbit, & Sobel, 1997) found that programs with more intense services were associated with higher levels of improvement in clinical, psychosocial and role functioning. The sample included 172 outpatients diagnosed with schizophrenia who were followed for 36 months. The Role Functioning Scale (Goodman, Sewell, Cooley, & Leavitt, 1993) was used to assess changes in the outpatients' role functioning.

In summary, the development of roles is a complex, lifelong process. Schizophrenia is a devastating mental illness impacting all areas of an individual's life. Learning of roles can be severely disrupted in an individual diagnosed with schizophrenia. As a result, individuals diagnosed with schizophrenia have often learned more passive, dependent roles than the active roles required in society today. Review of the literature indicates that some specialized programs have been developed to assist individuals diagnosed with schizophrenia in developing roles and their underlying skills.

THE DEVELOPMENT OF TASK
AND INTERPERSONAL SKILLS
IN RELATION TO ROLE DEVELOPMENT

The development of task and interpersonal skills has been viewed as an integral part of role satisfaction and manifestation (Kipper, 1991; Liberman et al., 1993). However, it is important that the development of task and interpersonal skills occurs within a larger meaningful context such as roles. Isolated skill development in the absence of a meaningful context is often viewed as ineffective and can lead to confusion and discouragement in therapy (Clark et al., 1997; Hocking, 2000).

An understanding of the importance of skill development within meaningful roles can be traced to Slagle (1924) and a program she developed on habit training (repetition of skills) to increase an individual's ability to live successfully in the community. Years later, Reilly (1962, 1969) emphasized the continuing need to address the neuromuscular, psychological and social skills that are the basic components of life's roles. Other authors corroborated that, in order to be successful in a variety of roles, one must be involved in "doing" the skills or components of these roles (Anthony, 1993; Fidler, 1969; Gutman, 1999; Jodrell & Sanson-Fisher, 1975; Liberman et al., 1993; Mosey, 1973; Smith & Tempone, 1968; Versluys, 1980; Wanderer, 1974).

In a review of outcome studies focused on skill development, skills have been directly or indirectly linked to the development of roles. For example, in directly linking skills to roles, one program developed groups that addressed skills of money management, personal grooming, and job seeking; the latter group specifically linked the skills of seeking gainful employment to the worker role (Broekema, Danz, & Schloemer, 1975). These groups incorporated both task and interpersonal skills. Versluys (1980) developed a variety of role-focused groups to develop social and interpersonal skills required for the development and maintenance of adult roles.

Other outcome studies had a less overt link between skills and roles. Some authors concluded that, for individuals with chronic mental illness, participation in skill-building programs is associated with positive rehabilitation outcomes, and that relapse frequencies for individuals who received skill training in addition to medication were consistently lower than for individuals who received medication alone (Anthony & Margules, 1974; Dion & Anthony, 1987; Mojtabai, Nicholson, & Carpenter, 1998). Several other authors designed programs aimed specifically at developing skills in individuals with chronic illnesses including schizophrenia (Goldstein, Gershaw, & Sprafkin, 1979; Lillie & Armstrong, 1982). Liberman et al. (1993) developed a series of training modules to address skill areas such as medication management, recreation and leisure, and personal hygiene. However, a direct link between skills and roles was not specifically mentioned in these studies.

Although some of the programs described were developed a few decades ago when hospital stays were lengthy and current medical (e.g., atypical psychotropic medications) and non-medical treatments were unavailable, the need for adequate task and interpersonal skills within roles is still apparent today (Lehman & Steinwachs, 1998; Mann et al., 1993). With the need to address skill development as soon as possible in treatment, Mann et al. (1993) developed a skills training program on an acute psychiatric unit to increase preparedness for community roles and to decrease recidivism. The groups in this program were designed to meet on a daily basis and participants joined the group as soon as feasible after admission.

Although much attention is given to the underlying social skills necessary for all roles, Fine (1994) viewed cognitive skills as the core of all task and social performances. In fact, it is her belief that social skill deficits are often the manifestation of basic underlying cognitive deficits. She asserted that problems, such as attention deficits, may produce a tendency to drift from the topic of conversation and decrease one's awareness of the verbal and nonverbal reactions of others. To address this problem she developed a program that addressed information processing, self-monitoring capacities and social-interpersonal skills in one-to-one and group formats.

In summary, task and interpersonal skills are the foundation of all roles. Because these skills may be undeveloped or underdeveloped in individuals diagnosed with schizophrenia, programs have been developed to teach these skills. Skill development programs have adapted to the changing mental health system, and skill training is still vital today. However, it is also important that skills are taught within a meaningful context, such as social roles. Role Development is designed to develop roles and the skills nested within these roles.

THE DEVELOPMENT AND DOCUMENTED USE
OF ROLE DEVELOPMENT

The primary source for Role Development (Schindler, 2002) is a set of guidelines for practice entitled Role Acquisition: An Acquisitional Frame of Reference (Mosey, 1986). In her discussion of acquisitional frames of reference, Mosey (1986) discussed three frames of reference contributing to the Role Acquisition frame of reference: action-consequence, activities therapy, and occupational behavior.

Action-Consequence is a frame of reference (Mosey, 1970) based on operant conditioning that addresses the areas of activities of daily living (ADL), avocational pursuits, and work. This frame of reference provides a link between learning theory and practice. Its evaluation procedures and postulates regarding change address the task skills and interpersonal relations required for success in the areas of ADL, avocational pursuits, and work.

Activities Therapy (Mosey, 1973) is a frame of reference that has a broader theoretical base than Action-Consequence and addresses three continuums: basic skills (task and group interaction skills); the public self (ADL, work, recreation, and intimacy); and the private self (cognitive system). It introduces the use of the teaching-learning process in intervention and the impact of group dynamics and processes on individual treatment. The facilitation of learning described by Bruner (1966) is evident. Concepts such as stimulating learning through curiosity, sustaining interest in learning through a sense of competence, using structured, meaningful tasks and having an astute, capable therapist as a teacher are integral parts of the teaching-learning process.

The Occupational Behavior frame of reference began with the early works of Reilly (1962, 1969) and was further developed by Kielhofner and Burke (1985) and Kielhofner (1995, 2002). This frame of reference originally emphasized the importance of play in exploring and understanding one's environment and described the individual as an open system with learning taking place through a continual process of input, throughput, output, and feedback. This process resulted in patterns of adaptive or maladaptive behavior. As work on this frame of reference progressed, the name was changed from Occupational Behavior frame of reference to the Model of Human Occupation. This frame of reference later expanded the role of throughput by dividing it into three subsystems: volition, habituation, and mind-brain-body performance. Roles and habits comprise the habituation subsystem whereas skills are addressed in the mind-brain-body performance subsystem. A current description of this frame of reference continues to include volitional processes, habituation, and performance capacities with a continuing appreciation for the impact of environment on occupations and the need for this intervention to occur within a client-centered approach (Kielhofner, 2002).

Role Development (Schindler, 2002) was developed specifically for the population under investigation. However, as mentioned earlier, the primary source for Role Development is the Role Acquisition frame of reference (Mosey, 1986). Although only one publication was found that directly addressed or examined the Role Acquisition frame of reference (Schindler, Connor, & Griffiths, 1995), two other publications (Custer & Wassink, 1991; Lyons & Morse, 1998) support the use of role development as an intervention.

A conference abstract (Schindler, Connor, & Griffiths, 1995) described the Role Acquisition frame of reference as the intervention used with an unemployed, 36-year-old male who was diagnosed with schizophrenia and committed to a forensic facility. The authors stated that through participation in a variety of occupational therapy groups, the patient was able to develop the task and interpersonal skills necessary to obtain a patient worker position in the facility and eventually a job in the community.

Custer and Wassink (1991) described an intervention in which they addressed social, vocational, and temporal adaptation skills with an individual diagnosed with major depression in preparation for a return to a student and eventually a worker role in broadcasting. Treatment addressed improvement of skills within a worker role.

Lyons and Morse (1988) developed an eight-phase work program to address the task, interpersonal and functional living skills required for success in all occupations. Participants progressed through treatment that included therapeutic work groups and supervised work placements. A subsequent evaluation of this program found that 79% of the patients who completed the program returned to work. This work program operated in an ambulatory care setting and assessed and developed prevocational skills in adults with head injuries.

Role Development, the set of guidelines for practice under investigation, is based primarily on the Role Acquisition frame of reference. To better meet the needs of the patients in this study, the Role Acquisition frame of reference was modified, resulting in Role Development. Role Acquisition evolved over 16 years as the author (Mosey, 1986) continued to expand on the behavioral framework and incorporate the work of other theorists. Although a few authors have apparently used interventions based on role performance in their treatment, there is no empirical information on Role Development or the Role Acquisition frame of reference.

CONCLUSION

This literature review has focused on four areas central to the topic: role theory, the development of roles in individuals diagnosed with schizophrenic disorders, the development of task and interpersonal skills in relation to the development of roles, and the development and documented use of Role Development. Role theory has evolved over 60 years in response to cultural and societal changes. Although the development of roles is typically a normal developmental process, this process can be extremely difficult for individuals diagnosed with schizophrenia. Because task and interpersonal skills are the foundation of roles, the learning and acquisition of these skills may also be limited for individuals diagnosed with schizophrenia. Role Development was designed to assist individuals diagnosed with schizophrenia to learn task and interpersonal skills within social roles. Although there is documented clinical use for this set of guidelines for practice, there is no empirical information to date that measures the effectiveness of the intervention.

Chapter 3

Role Development:
Treatment Guidelines

The intervention used in this study to assist individuals diagnosed with schizophrenia to develop social roles, and the task and interpersonal skills nested within these roles, is based on a set of guidelines for clinical practice entitled Role Development (Schindler, 2002). The format and foundation of this set of guidelines is based primarily on a modification of a set of guidelines for clinical practice entitled Role Acquisition: An Acquisitional Frame of Reference (Mosey, 1986). However, a comprehensive review of the literature on role theory, roles, and skills was conducted and pertinent information was incorporated into the development of this set of guidelines for practice. Role Development is designed for individuals who have not developed social roles, who have lost their social roles, or who wish to further develop their social roles. This set of guidelines addresses the development of task and interpersonal skills as they relate to an individual's roles as worker, student, group member, and friend.

An individual's social roles are usually more extensive than those mentioned above and often include roles as family member or community member. However, this study was conducted in a maximum-security psychiatric facility, in which the development of some roles is not feasible. For example, individuals in this setting are physically removed from family members throughout their hospitalization. Visits can occur

Note. This chapter is adapted from *Psychosocial Components of Occupational Therapy,* by A. C. Mosey, 1986, New York: Raven Press. Copyright 1986 by Raven Press. Adapted with permission.

[Haworth co-indexing entry note]: "Role Development: Treatment Guidelines." Schindler, Victoria P. Co-published simultaneously in *Occupational Therapy in Mental Health* (The Haworth Press, Inc.) Vol. 20, No. 3/4, 2004, pp. 25-45; and: *Occupational Therapy in Forensic Psychiatry: Role Development and Schizophrenia* (Victoria P. Schindler) The Haworth Press, Inc., 2004, pp. 25-45. Single or multiple copies of this article are available for a fee from The Haworth Document Delivery Service [1-800-HAWORTH, 9:00 a.m. - 5:00 p.m. (EST). E-mail address: docdelivery@haworthpress.com].

only at designated times and are often conducted through a glass window and via a telephone. Under these conditions it is difficult to develop a family role. Also, in this setting, individuals are unable to develop community roles because they have no access to the community. However, friend roles and group member roles may temporarily replace family and community roles. Therefore, this set of guidelines has been developed to address the needs of this population by addressing an individual's task and interpersonal skills within the roles of worker, student, group member, and friend.

GENERAL DESCRIPTION OF A SET OF GUIDELINES FOR PRACTICE

A set of guidelines for practice is a linking structure between theory and practice that organizes and applies information in order to achieve expected outcomes or goals. A set of guidelines for practice provides direction for problem identification (i.e., evaluation) and problem remediation (i.e., intervention) of a specific clinical condition. Sets of guidelines for practice have four components: (1) theoretical base; (2) function-dysfunction continuums; (3) behaviors indicative of function and dysfunction; and (4) postulates to promote positive change (Mosey, 1986, 1996).

The theoretical base of a set of guidelines for practice identifies the parameters of the set of guidelines and is the foundation from which all other parts of the set of guidelines are produced. It provides a rationale for describing and identifying function and dysfunction within the set of guidelines. It is derived from one or more theories. It may contain a static theory (one that describes relationships between phenomena but does not describe a process for change) but always contains a dynamic theory (a theory that describes a process for change) (Mosey, 1986, 1996).

Function/dysfunction continuums describe the area of human function associated with the set of guidelines for practice. A continuum represents a gradation from total inability to complete mastery of the function. In a continuum there is no absolute line or point that separates function and dysfunction, only a gradual increase or decrease in one's level of functioning in that particular area of function. Function-dysfunction continuums are deduced from the theoretical base; a set of guidelines for practice may have one or several function-dysfunction continuums (Mosey 1986, 1996).

Behaviors indicative of function and dysfunction are those specific areas of human performance that are characteristic of performance or lack of performance within that set of guidelines. These behaviors serve as a list of areas to identify in an evaluation process as present or absent, and form the framework for developing activities to be used in the evaluation process (Mosey, 1986, 1996).

Postulates to promote positive change are statements that delineate the way in which one assists an individual to move from a state of dysfunction to one of function. They serve as guides to the staff in designing the characteristics of the activities and the environment that are necessary to effect change (Mosey, 1986, 1996).

The following is a description of the four components that comprise the Role Development set of guidelines for practice used in this study: (1) theoretical base; (2) function-dysfunction continuums; (3) behaviors indicative of function and dysfunction; and (4) postulates to promote positive change (Mosey, 1986, 1996).

Theoretical Base

The theoretical concepts for the Role Development set of guidelines for practice were derived primarily from the Role Acquisition frame of reference (Mosey, 1986). A primary source for the theoretical base of the Role Acquisition frame of reference is social learning theory (Bandura, 1977). The theoretical base of Role Development addresses five principles: (1) the nature of the individual; (2) what needs to be learned; (3) how learning takes place; (4) typical and atypical development; and (5) appropriate tools.

The nature of the individual. All individuals have an inherent need to explore their environment and to experience a sense of competency and mastery in various aspects of daily living. This is especially true in aspects of the environment that are of interest to the individual. These interests develop from exploration and from the amount of worth placed on them by the individual's family and cultural group (Kielhofner, 1985, 1995, 2002; Mosey, 1986).

What needs to be learned. An individual's societal group and cultural orientation specify what one learns and categorizes into social roles (Durkheim, 1938; Mead, 1964). An individual's interests and goals also influence roles. Skill competence also has been viewed as an integral part of role satisfaction and manifestation (Heinssen, Liberman, & Kopelowicz, 2000; Kipper, 1991; Liberman et al., 1993; Sarbin, 1954). The foundation of all roles is task skills and interpersonal skills. To enact a role effectively, individuals need a repertoire of task and interpersonal skills. Task skills are those skills that address one's sensorimotor, cognitive, and psychological functions as they relate to the completion of tasks. Task skills that are basic to roles include paying attention, following directions, and solving problems related to a task. Interpersonal skills are those skills that address one's cognitive, psychological, and social functions as they relate to interactions with others. Interpersonal skills basic to roles include initiating and sustaining a conversation, and expressing one's ideas and feelings. Task and interpersonal skills are learned and refined as one participates in social roles. The social roles one may learn in this set of guidelines for practice include worker, student, friend, and group member (Black, 1976; Mosey, 1986; Liberman et al., 1993; Versluys, 1980).

How learning takes place. Learning of task and interpersonal skills and social roles occurs according to two processes: (1) the socialization process; and (2) the application of the principles of learning. The socialization process describes the agent (s) and the setting that facilitate the learning of a role. The agent (s) is the individual(s) responsible for collaborating with the patient regarding what is to be learned, and then providing feedback, and rewarding positive growth. The agent can be a positive role model who consistently and clearly defines expectations, provides constructive feedback, and rewards positive growth, or a negative role model that neglects this process or engages in this process in a destructive or harmful manner. For example, a parent who gently and consistently teaches his/her child appropriate moral and societal values would be viewed as a positive agent. To the contrary, a parent who ignores or neglects these teachings or teaches them in a way that is contrary to society's norms (e.g., teaching a child that the use of illegal drugs is acceptable), would be viewed as a negative agent. The ideal settings for the learning of adequate socialization are settings in which relevant behavior is "elicited, evoked, required, and permitted" (Bandura, 1977; Mosey, 1986, p. 451; Parsons, 1951a; Sarbin, 1954).

In Role Development an agent is clearly a facilitator. As a facilitator, the agent adheres to several principles. First, the agent assumes that the individual has knowledge of his/her needs regarding roles and skills. The individual, in collaboration with the agent, sets the agenda for therapy. Secondly, the agent accepts the individual's report as relevant information. Hence it is of the utmost importance to develop a plan that incorporates the individual's stated desires, goals and feedback. The final assumption is that the agent does not promote change but creates an environment to facilitate change (Law, 1998; Liberman & Kopelowicz, 2002; Pollock & McColl, 1998).

Settings in the socialization process should provide enough stimulation to generate interest, and practice of skills should be encouraged. For example, an ideal setting is one that is safe and has enough activities and interactions to stimulate exploration, competency, and mastery. A setting that is deprived, unsanitary, or harmful is not conducive to learning (Mosey, 1986; Parsons, 1951b).

Learning also occurs through the use of the Principles of Learning. These principles are psychological tenets that serve as a foundation to learning. A summation of these principles is as follows: (1) learning is influenced by an individual's inherent capacities, age, sex, interests, culture, and motivation; (2) learning is more likely to occur when learning goals are set by the individual and when the individual understands what is to be learned and the rationale for learning; (3) learning is increased when the individual is an active participant in learning and when learning begins at the individual's current level and proceeds at a comfortable rate; (4) frequent repetition, trial and error, reinforcement and feedback, and a supportive environment are important aspects of the learning process; and (5) anxiety affects learning differently, and conflicts and frustrations must be recognized and addressed (Mosey, 1986, p. 451).

Typical and atypical development. Typical development occurs when an individual interacts in an environment that promotes exploration, competency, and mastery. There are an adequate number of agents, and the agents are positive role models. The settings have an appropriate amount of stimulation and incentives to encourage the learning of social roles. The individual is motivated to explore and develop new roles in a satisfying manner. In atypical development, the number of agents may be inadequate and/or some of the agents may be unable or unwilling to encourage appropriate learning. Settings may be deprived or harmful. Atypical development could also occur due to a major life disruption such as illness or the loss of a role partner (Mosey, 1986; Parsons, 1951b).

Typically, the learning of roles follows a normal developmental progression (Black, 1976; Matsutsuyu, 1971; Thoits, 1983). This typical development of roles can become severely hindered by a diagnosis of mental illness. The more disabling the mental illness, the more it impacts on the learning of social roles. One of the most severe types of mental illness is one that encompasses schizophrenic disorders (Anthony, 1993; Pearlin, 1983; Shannon, 1972; Wessen, 1965). Instead of progressing through the typical development of roles and skills, many individuals diagnosed with schizophrenic disorders learn roles that are deviant or passive in nature and do not promote independent functioning in the community (Dickerson & Oakley, 1985; Gove & Lubach, 1968; Heard, 1977; Karmel, 1970; Pearlin, 1983; Shannon, 1972; Susser, Stein, Mountey, & Freeman, 1970; Versluys, 1980).

Appropriate tools. The tools used to evaluate performance and promote change in this set of guidelines for practice include the nonhuman environment (i.e., everything in an environment other than the individuals), conscious use of self (i.e., the staff's use of him/herself as a therapeutic tool), the teaching-learning process (teaching activities required for independent living), purposeful activities, activity analysis and synthesis (the process of developing, examining and selecting suitable activities), group dynamics, therapeutic groups, and activity groups. Within this set of guidelines for practice, tools should emphasize active participation in activities as opposed to passive participation or random activity. Activities should be real and tangible as opposed to abstract. In order to be successful in a variety of roles, one must be involved in "doing" the skills or components of these roles (Anthony, 1993; Fidler, 1969; Liberman et al., 1993; Mosey, 1973, 1986; Smith & Tempone, 1968; Versluys, 1980; Wanderer, 1974).

Function/Dysfunction Continuums

This set of guidelines for practice describes two categories of function/dysfunction continuums. They include Skills and Social Roles. Skills are: (1) task skills; and (2) interpersonal skills. The Skills involve coordination among an individual's motor, sensory/perception, cognitive, psychological, and social functions. Social Roles are: (1) worker; (2) student; (3) group member; and (4) friend. The task skills and interpersonal skills are necessary components for participation in social roles (Mosey, 1986).

Behaviors Indicative of Function and Dysfunction

The continuums are described in relation to behaviors indicative of dysfunction. The absence of these behaviors indicates function. These continuums consist of the two extremes of the continuum function and dysfunction. Intermediate stages of the continuum are not included between the two polarities of function and dysfunction. The categories and continuums are adapted from Mosey (1986) and Rogers, Sciarappa, and Anthony (1991) and are as follows (see Table 1).

TABLE 1. Function-Dysfunction Continuums

Task Skills	
1. Willingness to engage in doing tasks.	Avoids engaging in tasks, talks more than engages in productive activity, needs prompting or encouragement to engage in task, seems fearful when engaging in tasks.
2. Physical capacity (includes posture, strength, and gross and fine motor coordination).	Is unable to assume and/or maintain a posture that is conducive to successful completion of the task, tires very easily and/or asks for or takes an inordinate number of rest periods, clumsy carrying out tasks and/or performs tasks very slowly because of need to concentrate on coordinated movements.
3. Ability to maintain concentration on task.	Short attention span, spends most of the time engaged in nontask-oriented behavior (e.g., walking around), frequently changes tasks, leaves tasks uncompleted.
4. Ability to organize task in a logical manner.	Appears not to think about task prior to beginning, does not have all the items needed for task completion close at hand, does not consider what should be done first, second, and so forth.
5. Ability to follow directions.	Unable to comprehend directions, unable to follow directions without assistance, repeatedly asks for directions when these have been given and/or when available, does not return to directions to check whether the task is being done correctly.
6. Rate of performance.	Unable to work at a steady pace, is excessively slow in performing a task so that little is accomplished in comparison to others, or is excessively fast so that quality is sacrificed, spends considerable time on tasks but is not productive.
7. Attention to detail.	Excessive attention to detail, is not certain what aspects of a task are more or less important, conversely there may be excessive disregard of details, hurries through tasks with little attention to details.
8. Tolerates frustration.	Becomes upset when confronted with a problem, has difficulty in accepting delays, becomes agitated when he or she makes a mistake, has difficulty in accepting negative feedback, does not like to repeat steps or to do something again.

TABLE 1 (continued)

Interpersonal Skills

1. Ability to initiate, respond to, and sustain verbal interactions.

Has difficulty in spontaneously initiating a conversation with another person, does not spontaneously respond to others, cannot carry on a conversation, is not able to participate in normal give-and-take of conversation.

2. Keeps all statements appropriate to context.

Cannot follow thread of discussion, makes statements that are inappropriate or irrelevant to subject matter, is unable to keep statements appropriate despite redirection.

3. Communicates accurately and expresses self clearly.

Does not communicate in a way that is sensible to the listener, communicates false statements, expresses ideas in a circuitous or tangential manner.

4. Interacts comfortably with staff.

Is overly shy, friendly or in need of constant attention from staff, is not able to request or receive assistance from staff, is not able to follow direction, rules, or procedures from staff.

5. Interacts comfortably with peers.

Is overly shy, aggressive, or inappropriate with peers, acts as though he or she has not considered the needs or feelings of others, is not able to work collaboratively with peers, is not able to accept help from peers.

6. Uses appropriate non-verbal behavior and tone of voice.

Invades the space of others, tone of voice and/or non-verbal gestures are inconsistent or inappropriate to verbal content or context of the situation.

7. Cooperates as a member of a group.

Avoids interacting in groups, acts independently in situations where cooperation is required, treats cooperative situations as if they were competitive, has difficulty being the winner or the loser in a competitive group situation.

8. Controls impulsive, offensive, and/or annoying behavior.

Hastily acts out toward self or others in a negative or harmful manner, intentionally irritates, torments, teases, or causes anguish to others, is verbally degrading or abusive to others.

School Roles

1. Class attendance.

Frequently does not go to class, does not attend all classes, is late for and/or leaves early from class.

2. Group behavior.

Does not pay attention, disturbs other students, does not do tasks, does not participate in discussions.

32

3. Relationship with teachers.

Does not want to do what the teacher asks, ignores or is insolent to teacher, does not ask for guidelines or assistance when needed, cannot adapt to the style of some teachers, or is overly dependent on teacher.

4. Relationship with classmates.

States that he or she has no friends in class, is excessively shy with classmates, is a loner, or provokes classmates, acts as if superior to others, is not liked by classmates.

5. Academic performance.

Grades are below what one would expect given the individual's apparent abilities, grades are markedly uneven across subjects and/or grading periods, does not seem to put forth much effort, blames poor academic performance on others.

6. Participation in academic evaluations.

Does not study adequately for tests, hurries through examinations without giving appropriate attention to each item, or becomes excessively anxious prior to or during test, is overly preoccupied with grades.

Work

1. Attendance.

Attendance at work is irregular, frequently late to work, leaves work early, has difficulty tolerating a full session of work.

2. General attitude.

Does not feel the role of worker is an important social role, does not see self as a worker, is happier when not working.

3. Performance.

Manifests fear or anxiety as a response to the demand to be productive, does not organize tasks relative to priority, does not work at increased speeds when required, does not easily return to work after interruptions, does not plan work periods so that required amount of work is accomplished, avoids responsibility, does not complete assigned tasks in an acceptable manner, completes assigned tasks late.

4. Take direction from work supervisor.

Acts in a hostile or aggressive manner when assigned work, does not follow directions given, unable to accept constructive criticism, or is overly dependent on supervisor.

5. Relationship to co-workers.

Is overly dependent, does not give assistance when requested, is unable to carry on a casual conversation with co-workers, responds to co-workers in a belligerent manner, makes derogatory remarks to co-workers, avoids co-workers during breaks and lunch hour, acts in a way that makes co-workers uncomfortable.

6. Response to norms of the work setting.

Does not dress appropriately, selects inappropriate topics of conversation, pace of work is markedly different from workers, acts as if the work setting is designed to suit needs that are more appropriately satisfied in other settings, does not conform to the rules of the setting, cannot differentiate between formal and informal structure.

TABLE 1 (continued)

Group Membership

1. Group attendance.

Frequently does not go to group, does not attend all group sessions, is late for and/or leaves early from group sessions.

2. Group behavior.

Does not pay attention, disturbs other group members, does not do tasks, does not participate in discussions.

3. Relationship with group leaders.

Does not want to do what the group leader asks, ignores or is insolent to group leader, does not ask for guidelines or assistance when needed, cannot adapt to the style of some group leaders, or, is overly dependent on group leader.

4. Relationship with group members.

States that he or she has no friends in group, is excessively shy, avoids others during breaks, is unable to carry on a casual conversation, does not give assistance when requested, responds to others in a belligerent manner, makes derogatory remarks, acts as if superior to others, is not liked by group members.

5. Performance.

Manifests fear or anxiety as a response to the demand to be productive, does not organize tasks relative to priority, does not work at increased speeds when required, does not easily return to work after interruptions, does not plan work periods so that required amount of work is accomplished, avoids responsibility, does not complete assigned tasks in an acceptable manner, completes assigned tasks late.

6. Response to norms of the setting.

Does not dress appropriately, selects inappropriate topics of conversation, pace of task completion is markedly different from peers, does not conform to the rules of the setting.

Friendships

1. Initiates friendships.

States that he or she has no friends, does not know how to go about establishing friend relationships, states that there is no one that he or she can talk to.

2. Maintains friendships.

Spends little if any time with other people outside of the context of school/work/groups, has friendships for only a short period of time.

Postulates to Promote Positive Change (Mosey, 1986)

General Postulates to Promote Positive Change

- Long-term goals are based on the patient's expected environment.
- Task and interpersonal skills are developed within the context of social roles.
- A meaningful repertoire of behaviors is acquired through activities and interactions that (a) facilitate the relevant behavior; (b) are interesting to the individual and allow for exploration and movement toward mastery; (c) include role models; and (d) apply the principles of learning.
- It is best to use activities that are structured with an evident end product. Such activities tend to facilitate the desired behavior and the organization of behavior into useful patterns. They also provide a gauge for measuring progress of group members.
- There are several methods staff can use to facilitate desired behavior. Some of the methods are: (1) simply wait for the approximation of a desirable behavior and then reinforce that behavior; (2) encourage the patient to imitate another group member who is functioning fairly well in the group; (3) suggest to the patient (and encourage members of the group to do the same) that he or she try to act in a particular way, giving ideas about what the patient might say and do; (4) encourage trial-and-error interactions, with the patient receiving feedback about the appropriateness of experimental behavior; (5) have the group members pause periodically in their activity to examine what behavior has been useful to the group and to the individual, and what behavior has been harmful or of minimal use to the group and the individual. This process both reinforces the learning of appropriate behavior and gives group members clues as to the kinds of behavior that they might try. A discussion of this kind is kept as nonpersonal as possible. Group members are not singled out and told they did something right or wrong. Although immediate examples of what is occurring in the group are used, the discussion is oriented to talking about what kind of behavior is useful and what is not; (6) organize role-playing experiences. These may center around an incident that has recently occurred in the group or on a general problem area that several of the group members have in common (see also Table 2).

TABLE 2. Specific Postulates to Promote Positive Change

Task Skills	1. Willingness to engage in doing tasks.
	2. Physical capacity (includes posture, strength, and gross and fine motor coordination).
	3. Ability to maintain concentration on task.
	4. Ability to organize task in a logical manner.
	5. Ability to follow directions.
	6. Rate of performance.
	7. Attention to detail.
	8. Tolerates frustration.
Interpersonal Skills	1. Ability to initiate, respond to, and sustain verbal interactions.
	2. Keeps all statements appropriate to context.
	3. Communicates accurately and expresses self clearly.
	4. Interacts comfortably with staff.
	5. Interacts comfortably with peers.
	6. Uses appropriate non-verbal behavior and tone of voice.
	7. Cooperates as a member of a group.
	8. Controls impulsive, offensive, and/or annoying behavior.
School	1. Class attendance.
	2. Group behavior.
	3. Relationship with teachers.
	4. Relationship with classmates.
	5. Academic performance.
	6. Participation in academic evaluations.
Work	1. Attendance.
	2. General attitude.
	3. Performance.
	4. Take direction from work supervisor.
	5. Relationship to co-workers.
	6. Response to norms of the work setting.
Group Membership	1. Group attendance.
	2. Group behavior.
	3. Relationship with group leaders.
	4. Relationship with group members.
	5. Performance.
	6. Response to norms of the setting.
Friendships	1. Initiates friendships.
	2. Maintains friendships.

Specific Postulates to Promote Positive Change

Task Skills

1. Willingness to Engage in Doing Tasks

Patients who have difficulty in doing simple tasks need frequent, clear, and non-judgmental support and encouragement. Frequently staff must spend considerable time establishing a relationship of trust between him or herself and the patient. The patient may feel that other people do not understand how difficult it is for him or her to do anything that requires overt, self-initiated action. Learning is enhanced if the patient and staff mutually share the initial tasks. Later staff might introduce tasks in which the patient does one part independently while staff does another part. Finally, the patient is encouraged to do simple tasks alone. For patients who avoid participating in tasks because of fear of being judged, the change process is initiated with tasks where there are few measurable standards; it then moves to tasks that require self-judgment, and to tasks that can be judged by some measurable external standard.

2. Physical Capacity

Staff demonstrates and, if necessary, helps the patient to take appropriate postures for various tasks. If the patient is unable to take an adequate posture because of physical limitations, staff helps the patient take the best possible position and/or makes adaptations in the activity. Staff grades activities relative to strength required and length of time of involvement in activities. Initially, frequent rest periods are scheduled with these diminishing over time. Staff grades activities relative to the need for gross and fine-motor movements. If the patient has difficulty in both areas, gross coordination is given attention first.

3. Ability to Maintain Concentration on Task

To help a patient increase attention span, staff and the patient decide how long the patient will work without interruption. Initially, this may be a very short period of time. Just being able to engage in a task for a limited period of time may be sufficiently reinforcing, or staff may have to provide some additional reinforcement. The length of the work period is slowly increased at a rate that is comfortable for the patient. Sometimes patients do not complete projects because they select ones that take a very long time to complete, or they are too complex or too repetitive for them. Thus, in the beginning of the change process, the patient is helped to choose a task that is relatively short-term and fairly easy to do. As the change process progresses, the patient is encouraged to select tasks that take an increasingly longer time to complete and are increasingly more complex.

4. Ability to Organize Task in a Logical Manner

Patients who have difficulty in this area are helped to think about a task before it is begun. They are encouraged to consider the amount of time that will be needed, to locate all the items they will need for task completion, and to consider what should be done first, second, and so on. Activities are presented in a graded manner relative to the degree of organization required and the cognitive level of the patient.

5. Ability to Follow Directions

Patients who have difficulty following directions may not be able to follow one particular type of instruction (e.g., oral, demonstrated, pictorial, or written). A type of direction that the patient is able to follow is offered. For example, a patient may understand how to do a task only if shown how; verbal directions are not sufficient. The change process would begin with staff instructing the patient on how to do the activity and demonstrating the activity at the same time. On the other hand, some patients are able to follow only one-step instructions. When that is the case, the change process begins at that level. Staff slowly increases the number of steps given with directions one at a time.

6. Rate of Performance

When a patient works too slowly, a short time limit is set in the initial stages of the change process. This may be as little as three minutes. The patient is asked to complete a part of the task that takes a specific period of time to do when it is done at a normal rate. If the patient does not finish the task, a shorter time period is set. The patient is allowed to rest for a few minutes and then is asked to work for the specified time again, and so on until the task is finished. Time periods for subsequent tasks are slowly increased in length. Activities should be short-term, allowing the patient to complete an activity in one session. This helps the patient to experience a sense of accomplishment. When a patient works too fast, causing errors in the task, he is encouraged to identify the errors and to decrease his speed.

7. Attention to Detail

Patients who give excessive attention to detail need to be encouraged to be a little less detail-oriented, or to leave something undone or undone for the time being. The patient is likely to need a considerable amount of reinforcement and reassurance that nothing horrible is going to happen if something is not done perfectly. Patients who do not give sufficient attention to detail essentially need the opposite approach. Details they miss should be pointed out. Positive reinforcement is given when the patient goes back and corrects an error and when the patient does a task in which the majority of the details are taken into consideration.

8. Tolerates Frustration

It is important that staff be aware of what kinds of situations frustrate the patient. With this knowledge, staff is able to grade activities so that initially the patient is presented with minimal sources of frustration. Gradually the patient is introduced to activities that are potentially more frustrating. The patient is given suggestions about alternative and more adaptive ways of dealing with frustrating solutions. Positive reinforcement is given when the patient deals adequately with a potentially frustrating situation.

Interpersonal Skills

Specific postulates regarding change for interpersonal skills are:

1. Ability to Initiate, Respond to, and Sustain Verbal Interactions

The staff initially reinforces nonverbal responses but diminishes such reinforcement over time, with the major reinforcement being given to verbal behavior. Activities requiring little verbal interaction may be used at the beginning of the change process with gradation toward activities that require more verbal interaction. If at all possible, patients with difficulties in this area should be placed in groups where some group members have at least partially mastered this skill. This provides an opportunity for adequate role models.

2. Keeps All Statements Appropriate to Context

For patients who make statements that are inappropriate or irrelevant to current subject matter, staff assists the patient in understanding that the statement does not apply to the group topic and encourages the expression of statements that are relevant. Staff may suggest that the patient observe another patient who is modeling the appropriate behavior, or staff may suggest relevant topics to which the patient can provide a comment.

3. Communicates Accurately and Expresses Self Clearly

For patients who do not communicate in a way that is understandable to the listener, staff assists the patient in restating his/her thought and encourages the patient to ask the listener(s) for feedback concerning the communication. For patients who make false statements or express ideas in a circuitous or tangential manner, staff encourages the patient to examine his communication, ask the group for feedback, and determine how he/she would like to change the statement or adhere more closely to the topic.

4. Interacts Comfortably with Staff

Individuals with difficulty in this area need to be supported in understanding that staff is there to help them. Through appropriate verbal and non-verbal interactions, staff will convey a sense of comfort to the patients. For patients who are overly shy, friendly or in need of constant attention in interactions with staff, staff can gently but consistently provide assistance or set limits depending on the need of the situation.

5. Interacts Comfortably with Peers

For patients who are aggressive or inappropriate in interactions with peers, staff must first ensure that the group situation is safe and therapeutic. Patients who have not considered the needs or feelings of others, act as though one's own needs or feelings are always paramount, or are not able to work collaboratively with peers, must receive consistent and firm feedback about the negative consequences of this behavior. Once the patient is aware of this, the learning of more appropriate behaviors can occur via role playing and modeling. Patients who are overly shy and not able to accept help from peers need an environment that is safe and comfortable and will allow them to practice communicating with peers in a way that is supported by staff.

6. Uses Appropriate Non-Verbal Behavior and Tone of Voice

For patients who invade the space of others, make gestures, or use a tone of voice (e.g., loud) that is inappropriate for the group, staff must first act to ensure that the group is safe. Patients who have become threatening or assaultive will need to be escorted from the group. However, if a patient is beginning to demonstrate this type of behavior, staff can speak to the patient individually or ask the group to give the patient feedback about his behavior. Staff can ask the patient if he is aware of the change in his behavior and if he knows the reason for the change. Staff or group members can ask the patient if he understands the effect he is having on others in the group. Finally, staff or other patients can help the patient to identify more appropriate ways to interact. Patients who had to be escorted from the room can be involved in this same type of discussion when they are calm and open to feedback.

7. Cooperates as a Member of a Group

Initially staff selects activities requiring minimal cooperation. These may be fairly individualized activities in the context of a group. Activities are then graded so that increasingly more cooperative and/or competitive behavior is necessary. What is required for a cooperative venture is made very clear. After the first stages of the change process, it is recommended that the activity be designed so that success of the activity is dependent on adequate cooperation of those involved. Group members selecting and planning activities together frequently provide the necessary stimuli for facilitating the development of this skill. Regarding competition, patients often need assistance in learning how to win and lose in a "graceful" manner. Appropriate behavior as a winner or loser and toward a winner or loser is emphasized and reinforced. This is done with full acceptance of the feelings of the involved individuals.

8. Controls Impulsive, Offensive, and/or Annoying Behavior

Individuals with difficulty in this area may have little, if any, idea how their behavior affects other people. Such a deficit is primarily altered by feedback. The patient is assisted in identifying what he or she is doing and the effect of that behavior on others. The patient is helped to become "self-reflective" about behavior–to know essentially, "What am I doing now?" The patient is assisted in learning how to study the effects of actions. Another problem individuals have in this area is deficits in understanding rights and responsibilities relative to interpersonal relations. These should be made explicit by the staff and, if possible, other group members. Respect for the rights of others is reinforced.

School

The majority of patients admitted to a maximum-security psychiatric facility have had negative experiences with their school situations. Many of the patients were in special education classes and many had difficulty successfully obtaining a high school diploma. Very few have a college education.

For individuals who are under 22 years of age, formal classroom instruction is required by law. A classroom setting within a facility is structured so that the teacher is in an authority position and the individuals in the program are classmates. Both individual and group activities are used as vehicles for intervention. Within the context of these activities, the teacher, through the grading of activities, feedback, and reinforcement, helps the patient develop the task and interpersonal skills required for the role of student.

For older individuals, three areas of education have been identified (adult basic skills, adult education, and life issues). Adults who may not have mastered basic skills (reading, writing and math), may be interested in developing competency in this area. Adults interested in expanding their learning may do so in areas such as computer training. Also, although topics should be developed according to an individual's needs, group instruction on life issues (e.g., learning about mental illness, nutrition) may be relevant to many patients.

Regardless of the student's age or educational needs, students should be encouraged to develop the habits required for success in the role of student. Students are encouraged to arrive to class on time and to attend class consistently. Educational tasks are structured to stimulate a patient's interests and to provide the "just right challenge" to facilitate appropriate behaviors and academic performance. To facilitate appropriate relationships with teacher and classmates, formal rules and expectations of the class can be presented when the student begins in the program and reviewed as needed.

Work

Learning the role of worker is best accomplished in a situation that is a reasonable simulation of the demands of a realistic work environment. The opportunity must exist for the patient to experience the full range of interpersonal relationships, time demands, and basic skills that will be encountered in a work environment.

The majority of patients admitted to a maximum security psychiatric facility have little, if any, experience with work, and involvement in work was often short-term, unsuccessful, and in the distant past. Therefore, the ideal situation for intervention offers the patient an opportunity to develop skills first in the institution's sheltered workshop, and then, if appropriate, progress to a hospital job.

When a patient has acquired some very basic habits and is able to function in a group with a minimal number of personal difficulties, he or she can begin in a sheltered workshop. The sheltered workshop contains more people than a typical therapy group and the atmosphere is more work-oriented. The staff member is a foreman or a work supervisor and other patients may be assistant supervisors. For some patients, this will be their first experience of being paid for their work, and their amount of pay will depend upon the amount of work they produce.

Staff, in the role of supervisor, assigns tasks and gives adequate instruction as to how the tasks should be accomplished. Staff ensure that the patient can perform the work independently, but they still observe and supervise the patient as necessary. Emphasis is placed on accuracy, and doing the job at the rate that would be expected in competitive employment. Staff identifies problems, adjusts those conditions of work that will help the patient, and provides appropriate feedback and reinforcement while acting as a supervisor.

A patient is helped to overcome problems in interpersonal relations by assisting him/her in identifying the expectations of a work setting and how the patient's behavior is contrary to those expectations. More acceptable ways of interacting are suggested to the patient and he or she is urged to try out these suggestions. Staff and fellow patients (i.e., co-workers) provide support and reinforcement.

When a patient is functioning well in a sheltered workshop, he or she may progress to a hospital job. A hospital job is a part-time work assignment in the facility in areas such as the laundry, library, coffee shop, or in working as a rehabilitation assistant in one of the rehabilitation programs. The patient is given the same responsibilities and assignments that would be given to anyone in that position. The patient is also offered the usual coffee breaks and is given the opportunity to work without excess supervision. Pay is usually at minimum wage.

Hospital jobs provide the patient with an experience of a real work situation. She/he is able to observe other workers and compare behavior to their way of working and interacting. Thus the patient receives direct reinforcement for appropriate behavior on the job.

Group Membership

Patients may be involved in a variety of other groups in occupational therapy, recreation, or creative arts therapy. Goals within each of these groups will vary, but they all will promote the role of group member and development of task and interpersonal skills.

Both individual and group activities are used as vehicles for intervention. Within the context of these activities, staff, through the grading of activities, feedback, and reinforcement, helps the patient develop the task and interpersonal skills required for the role of a group member.

In these groups, interpersonal and task difficulties are identified. Group members are encouraged to develop ways to address one's own difficulties, and if appropriate, to offer constructive feedback to others. However, staff supervises this process and ensures that behaviors and feedback are productive and supportive. If behavioral problems occur, the corrective action plan similar to the one described for the school program is used.

Friendships

Prior to engaging in the development of skills necessary to form and maintain friendships, the patient must have some basic skills in interpersonal relationships. A person usually learns how to make friends by engaging in activities with friendly people and by observing how friends interact.

Some patients have had no experience in making friends. They do not know how to engage in conversation with another person or how to ask someone to join in an activity. In this case staff often needs to talk with the patient about what is involved in making and keeping friends. The patient is urged to spend time with other people with whom he would like to develop friendships.

Initially, the patient is encouraged to engage in activities with another person in the group. In this way staff can provide the necessary support to facilitate the development of a friendship. Once this is accomplished, the patient is encouraged to interact with others outside the structure of an organized activity (e.g., eating a meal with another patient on the unit). Staff support, advise, reassure, and arrange the situation so the patient receives positive reinforcement for interactions leading to the development of a friendship. This external reinforcement may be necessary until the patient receives internal reinforcement from participating in a successful friendship.

People also learn about friendships by observing how other friends act. Thus, spontaneous friendships are encouraged and staff who are friends are encouraged to act as role models for the patients.

Chapter 4

Implementing Role Development: Tools and Resources

To accurately implement Role Development (Schindler, 2002), the set of guidelines for practice, several issues are considered. First, it is imperative that the staff implementing the set of guidelines participate in adequate and effective training. The protocol for staff training is described below. Next, it is necessary to describe the way in which staff implement the set of guidelines for practice with the patients. Therefore, the following questions must be addressed: (1) What will staff say and do with the patients to implement the set of guidelines for practice? and (2) How will staff and patients work collaboratively to choose goals and activities for the patients? Finally, it is important to recognize that supervision, ongoing instruction, feedback, and support be continually provided to the staff to ensure that fidelity to the set of guidelines to practice is maintained. All of these items were included in the study described in this volume. The method for including these items is described below.

STAFF TRAINING

Because all of the rehabilitation staff involved in this study implemented both the multidisciplinary activity program and the Role Development program, the comparison and experimental groups occurred in a

---

[Haworth co-indexing entry note]: " Implementing Role Development: Tools and Resources." Schindler, Victoria P. Co-published simultaneously in *Occupational Therapy in Mental Health* (The Haworth Press, Inc.) Vol. 20, No. 3/4, 2004, pp. 47-56; and: *Occupational Therapy in Forensic Psychiatry: Role Development and Schizophrenia* (Victoria P. Schindler) The Haworth Press, Inc., 2004, pp. 47-56. Single or multiple copies of this article are available for a fee from The Haworth Document Delivery Service [1-800-HAWORTH, 9:00 a.m. - 5:00 p.m. (EST). E-mail address: docdelivery@haworthpress.com].

Digital Object Identifier: 10.1300/J004v20n03_04

sequential manner. Staff training occurred after the completion of the comparison group but prior to the initiation of the experimental group. In this way, staff were not influenced by the experimental intervention prior to its implementation. A total of 15.5 hours of formal training occurred followed by individual training. A staff training manual containing all of the information described below was developed and provided to each staff member. The training occurred as follows:

1. Assessment of Each Staff Member's Current Level of Understanding Regarding Role Functioning

To assess each staff member's current level of understanding regarding role functioning, a written case history of a patient residing in the facility (who met the criteria for the study) was given to each staff member. This case history included the patient's age, sex, diagnoses, psychiatric history, psychiatric problems warranting the current admission, current mental status, brief physical, family, social, and work history, and the results of the occupational therapy evaluation conducted on admission, including the patient's current strengths and needs. This information was provided because the same type of information was given to the staff on each patient participating in the study. Based on this information, each staff member was asked: (1) How would you set up treatment with this patient if you are trying to help him develop roles? (2) What skills would you identify as being important to the development of these roles? How would you and the patient work together to help him develop these roles and skills? (3) What goals would you set? (4) What activities would you choose to meet the goals? and (5) How would you prioritize and organize the patient's treatment? Once completed, staff members shared their plans with the group and subsequently gave these plans to the Principal Investigator (PI). The Principal Investigator used these plans to determine the staff's learning needs.

2. Didactic Instruction on Sets of Guidelines for Practice

General information regarding sets of guidelines for practice was provided such as: What is a set of guidelines for practice? What kinds of sets of guidelines for practice exist? Why use a set of guidelines for practice? To address these questions resources were used and information was summarized into written handouts (Miller & Walker, 1993; Mosey, 1996).

3. Didactic Instruction on the Set of Guidelines for Practice Used in This Study (i.e., Role Development Presented in Chapter 3)

Handouts and a PowerPoint presentation were used as instructional aides.

4. Group Case Study

A written case history was presented (same format as described in #1), but the entire group worked collaboratively (using the resources described in #3) to develop a treatment plan for the patient based on Role Development. The Principal Investigator reviewed the written plan and constructive feedback was provided.

5. Simulation of a Staff/Patient Interview and a Group Activity

The Principal Investigator simulated a staff/patient interview with a staff member enacting the role of a patient. Also, a group activity was simulated in which staff identified task and interpersonal skills and the roles within which these skills occur. Again, staff enacted roles of patients. Then, under the guidance of the Principal Investigator, staff identified the roles and skills that could be developed and designed strategies to achieve their development.

6. Small Group Case Study

Another written case history of a patient was distributed (same format as described in #1) to three staff groups (6-7 members each) and staff were instructed to develop a treatment plan for the patient based on Role Development. Each of these groups worked with a mentor and the resources described above. The mentors were the PI and two staff occupational therapists with several years of experience implementing sets of guidelines for practice. The mentors and the PI reviewed the treatment plans and constructive feedback was provided to each group.

7. Individual Case Study

Another written case history was distributed, with the same format as described in #1, to each staff member to develop a treatment plan for the patient based on Role Development. The mentors and the resources were available to each staff member. The mentor and the PI reviewed the treatment plan and constructive feedback was provided to each staff member.

8. Individual Homework/Posttest Assignment

Each staff member was asked to select a patient with whom he/she is currently working who would meet the criteria for the study. Using the case history method described above, each staff member was asked to formulate a case history and then develop a plan of intervention using the format outlined for the case study. The mentors and the PI reviewed the treatment plan and constructive feedback was provided.

9. Individual Staff Training

The Principal Investigator observed each staff member as he/she conducted a group session. Upon completion of the observation, the Principal Investigator and the staff member brainstormed methods for the staff member to implement Role Development with patients in his/her group.

STAFF IMPLEMENTATION OF THE SET OF GUIDELINES FOR PRACTICE WITH THE PATIENTS

All patients who met the criteria for the study and agreed to participate in the study were assigned to four one-hour rehabilitation groups/day. However, only the patients involved in the Role Development program participated in the process described below (see Appendix A, page 163–Role Development Study Procedures).

Once the patient's schedule was developed, the staff members leading the groups to which the patient was assigned were informed of the patient's participation in the study. Once the patient began his regularly scheduled programs, a rater observed and interviewed the patient and completed the four rating scales. A copy of the Role Checklist was forwarded to each group leader so that he/she was aware of the past, current, and future roles selected by the patient. The group leaders then conducted their own assessment of the patient, using forms derived from the function-dysfunction continuums, and established a baseline of functioning in the task skills and interpersonal skills because these skills are the starting point and foundation of all roles. Once the staff member completed the assessment, he/she referred to the function/dysfunction continuums of the set of guidelines for practice to determine the patient's strengths and needs in each of the continuums. The staff member focused only on those continuums relevant for that group. For example, a teacher with a patient in the education program focused on continuums of task skills, interpersonal skills, and the role(s) of student, and friend (if appropriate).

Once the staff member determined the patient's current level of functioning, he/she referred to the postulates to promote change to determine how to assist the patient. The postulates to promote positive change give the staff member a guideline in which to choose appropriate activities, facilitate the necessary interactions, and make the necessary modifications to the environment in order to promote change. All group leaders working with the patient participated in this process. Group leaders were encouraged to consult with each other and receive assistance from the PI so that fidelity to the set of guidelines for practice could be maintained.

Once the group leader ascertained the information described above, he/she met with the patient and reviewed this information. They reviewed the Role Checklist and prioritized the roles the patient selected to address and the roles that could realistically be addressed in that group. For example, the roles of worker and friend could be addressed in the Sheltered Workshop program but the role of student could not. The group leader and the patient discussed the types of typical activities and interactions that occur in the group, and together they chose the activities and interactions the patient participated in to develop the task and interpersonal skills that comprise the desired role (see Appendix B, pp. 165-175).

At least weekly, and more often if necessary, the group leader and the patient met for approximately 15 minutes to discuss the patient's progress with the treatment intervention. During the meeting the patient was asked questions such as:

Do you think you made progress toward developing your role this week?
If not, what got in the way of progress this week?
If so, what role(s) did you work on?
How did you work on this role(s)?
What activities helped you to work on this role?
What interactions helped you to work on this role?
What are your thoughts/feelings about the progress you made?
To continue making progress, what activities and interactions would you like to plan for next week?

If the patient was unable to identify progress or lack of progress, the group leader was prepared to identify and describe this for the patient. For example, if the patient wanted to develop the role of friend within a recreation group, and the patient participated in recreational games with two or three other patients in the last week, the group leader identified these situations for the patient. The group leader also gave the patient specific examples of his interactions with the other group members and described how these interactions are typical of interactions that friends have with one another. If the patient was unable to work on the relevant skills and roles, the group leader and the patient explored what occurred in the past week to limit progress. Together a plan was developed for the upcoming week.

The group leader consistently referred to the relevant function-dysfunction continuums and the postulates to promote positive change to monitor the patient's progress (or lack of progress) and to continually collaborate with the patient on choosing the activities, facilitating the interactions, and modifying the environment to promote positive change.

The process of referring to the set of guidelines for practice and weekly meetings with the patient continued throughout the patient's hospitalization or through the end of the study (whichever occurred first). At the time of the patient's discharge or the completion of the patient's participation in the study, an additional meeting was held with the patient to summarize the patient's progress and make long-term plans for the patient's continued involvement in developing roles in his life.

TREATMENT FIDELITY

Treatment fidelity is an important but relatively recent consideration in research. It concerns two related, but distinct issues. The first, which has also been referred to as treatment integrity or treatment adherence, concerns the degree to which a treatment intervention is implemented as intended and in a uniform manner. Treatment integrity can suffer over time. Program drift, a concept that refers to the negative impact of time on fidelity, occurs as implementers modify or omit program activities over time (Durlak, 1998; McGrew, Bond, Dietzen, & Salyers, 1994; Moncher & Prinz, 1991; Rice & Meyer, 1994; Scanlon, Horst, Nay, Schmidt, & Waller, 1977).

The second aspect of treatment fidelity, which has also been referred to as treatment differentiation, refers to the extent to which treatment conditions differ from one another so that the manipulation of the independent variable occurred as intended. Two treatment groups or treatment and control groups could be so similar that they are not seen as two distinct groups. Failure to adhere to treatment fidelity can lead to a Type III error or the measurement of something that does not exist. Failure to implement a treatment intervention as planned could lead to measuring something other than the treatment intervention. Since this "other" was not identified in the study, the researcher ends up measuring something that does not exist (Durlak, 1998; McGrew, Bond, Dietzen, & Salyers, 1994; Moncher & Prinz, 1991; Rice & Meyer, 1994; Scanlon, Horst, Nay, Schmidt, & Waller, 1977).

A review of 359 treatment outcome studies from major journals revealed that the majority of the studies (55%) ignored the issue of treatment fidelity. Sixty-three studies published between 1987-1996 found that the effect size associated with skills teaching is generally larger when the skills taught and the skills evaluated are highly similar. Although this suggests that learned material may not generalize to other situations in patients' lives, it does support the importance of fidelity in developing interventions and evaluating their effectiveness (Baronet & Gerber, 1998).

Fidelity is important to maintain internal and external validity. In internal validity, a study producing statistically significant results but failing to ensure fidelity leaves a question as to whether the treatment outcome was due to an effective treatment or to unknown contaminants added to the treatment. In external validity, treatment replication requires adequate documentation of treatment fidelity. Inadequate descriptions of the treatment intervention or of its implementation make it difficult to replicate the treatment. Fidelity also impacts statistical power. If fidelity is high, the probability of behavior change is also high, and sound methodology is highly correlated with effect size (Moncher & Prinz, 1991).

Treatment fidelity can be achieved if several factors are addressed. First, treatments must be adequately defined. Failure to operationalize treatments leads to ambiguity in the understanding and implementation of treatment. Clear definitions and specification of content and procedures are necessary to ensure that the active ingredient is being delivered (Moncher & Prinz, 1991). Also, the ideal intervention contains only those elements necessary to achieve desired goals (Durlak, 1998).

Comprehensive training is essential to ensure that the individuals delivering the treatment do not omit procedures or introduce unplanned procedures into the treatment. Clear written materials, didactic teaching, role-plays, and supervision of sessions promote fidelity (Moncher & Prinz, 1991). Training can also ease a therapist's uneasiness about implementing a new intervention by promoting a sense of comfort and preparedness with the new intervention. A study comparing trained and untrained teachers who taught health modules to adolescents found that trained teachers implemented the modules with a significantly higher degree of fidelity ($p = .025$), and knowledge scores were significantly higher for classes taught by trained teachers ($p < .001$) but not for classes taught by untrained teachers ($p < .075$) (Ross, Leupler, Nelson, Saavedra, & Hubbard, 1991). In another study, trainers' competency in teaching social and instrumental skills to patients with severe mental illness was measured by directly observing the trainers and determining the fidelity of their behaviors to those specified in the module's manual (Wallace, Liberman, MacKain, Blackwell, & Eckman, 1992).

Treatment manuals or comprehensive written materials reduce the variance in treatment administration. These resources guide and standardize the treatment implementation. However, some nuances of intervention, such as *how* something is said or done, may be more subtle and difficult to prescribe in manuals. In that case, customizing the intervention to fit the host setting and the target population is essential (Durlak, 1998).

Ongoing supervision of individuals delivering the treatment is essential to ensure accuracy. Even when trainees demonstrate competence in learning new interventions, there is little guarantee that they will use the skills once the training has ceased. In fact, researchers in one school-based study observed that although teachers would enthusiastically state that their lives and their teaching practice were dramatically changed as a result of learning a new teaching practice, upon observation, the teaching practice looked quite ordinary (Kauffman, 1996). Continual reinforcement is necessary. In the same way supervisors provide ongoing supervision to staff to maintain skills, and the instructors of the new intervention must continue to provide teaching and supervision to the professional and paraprofessional staff to maintain competent levels of behavioral intervention. Clinical supervision includes support and guidance, feedback and ongoing individualized training, and inspiration to continue to implement newly learned skills (Corrigan & Jakus, 1994). Weekly meetings, review of taped sessions, and role-playing can be part of the supervision process (Durlak, 1998).

In one study, another measure to ensure fidelity involved the leader of the group completing a fidelity measure after the group was completed. This measure tapped the leader's perceptions of session fidelity and effectiveness. Each component of the session was rated for fidelity. A limitation with this method is that the raters of fidelity are also the leaders of the group and could be biased in their reports. However, if raters other than the group leader also evaluate the session, the bias may be limited. Also, this form of rating fidelity could be carried out in addition to other measures of fidelity (Rice & Meyer, 1994).

FIDELITY TO THE SET OF GUIDELINES FOR PRACTICE

The foundation for building fidelity to the set of guidelines for practice began during staff training. Prior to initiation of the experimental intervention, staff demonstrated competency in implementing the set of guidelines for practice via the nine steps described earlier in the Staff Training section of this chapter.

Ongoing fidelity to the set of guidelines for practice was monitored via the following methods:

1. Biweekly observation by the Principal Investigator of staff/patient interviews followed by constructive feedback.
2. Biweekly observation of group sessions in which the staff member is implementing the set of guidelines for practice with one or more patients, e.g., staff and patient (s) are collaboratively choosing and implementing activities promoting the learning of predetermined roles.
3. Weekly meetings with all staff involved in the Role Development program to review each patient's progress.
4. Principal Investigator completed the Fidelity Checklist-PI (see Table 3) after observation of groups.
5. Staff member completed the Fidelity Checklist-Staff Member (see Table 4) after the Principal Investigator observed his/her group.

TABLE 3. Fidelity Checklist Forms

FIDELITY CHECKLIST FORM for STAFF COMPLIANCE
TO BE COMPLETED BY PRINCIPAL INVESTIGATOR

Item	Compliant	Non-compliant	N/A	Comments
Initial Session				
Staff met with patient upon initial attendance at group				
Staff reviewed Role Checklist with patient				
Staff and patient established roles to develop in group				
Staff and patient collaboratively chose activities to address roles				
Ongoing Sessions				
Staff meets individually with patient at least once weekly				
Staff discussed with patient his progress/lack of progress toward development of roles in past week				
Staff and patient collaboratively chose activities to promote specific role development				
Staff modified environment and facilitated interpersonal interactions to promote development of roles				
Staff and patient discussed plan of action (activities, environment) to promote role development in upcoming week				

TABLE 4. Fidelity Checklist Forms

FIDELITY CHECKLIST FORM for STAFF COMPLIANCE
TO BE COMPLETED BY STAFF MEMBER

Item	Compliant	Non-compliant	N/A	Comments
Initial Session				
I met with patient upon initial attendance at group				
I reviewed the Role Checklist with patient				
Patient and I established roles for him to develop in group				
Patient and I collaboratively chose activities to address roles				
Ongoing Sessions				
I meet individually with patient at least once weekly				
I discussed with patient his progress/lack of progress toward development of roles in past week				
I and the patient collaboratively chose activities to promote specific role development				
I modified the environment and facilitated interpersonal interactions to promote development of roles				
Patient and I discussed plan of action (activities, environment) to promote role development in upcoming week				

Chapter 5

Designing an Outcomes-Based Research Study to Assess the Development of Roles in Adults Diagnosed with Schizophrenia

The research problem in this study is to ascertain if adults diagnosed with schizophrenic disorders demonstrate improved task and interpersonal skills and social roles when involved in an individualized intervention based on the Role Development program (RDP), in comparison to an intervention based on a multidepartmental activity program (MAP). A pretest-posttest repeated measures design was used.

SAMPLE

This study was conducted at a maximum-security psychiatric facility. Six inclusion criteria were used: (1) age; (2) gender; (3) diagnosis; (4) participant ability to read and speak English; (5) length of stay; and (6) Global Assessment of Functioning (GAF) score (*DSM-IV-R*, 2000). Each of these criterion are described below.

Participants were adult males, 18-55 years of age, who have been diagnosed with a schizophrenic disorder. Schizophrenic disorders are

[Haworth co-indexing entry note]: "Designing an Outcomes-Based Research Study to Assess the Development of Roles in Adults Diagnosed with Schizophrenia." Schindler, Victoria P. Co-published simultaneously in *Occupational Therapy in Mental Health* (The Haworth Press, Inc.) Vol. 20, No. 3/4, 2004, pp. 57-77; and: *Occupational Therapy in Forensic Psychiatry: Role Development and Schizophrenia* (Victoria P. Schindler) The Haworth Press, Inc., 2004, pp. 57-77. Single or multiple copies of this article are available for a fee from The Haworth Document Delivery Service [1-800- HAWORTH, 9:00 a.m. - 5:00 p.m. (EST). E-mail address: docdelivery@haworthpress.com].

http://www.haworthpress.com/web/OTMH
Digital Object Identifier: 10.1300/J004v20n03_05

those disorders listed in the DSM-IV-R (*DSM-IV-R*, 2000) Axis I diagnosis of the patient's hospital record as schizophrenia, undifferentiated type (295.90); schizophrenia, residual type (295.60); schizophrenia, catatonic type (295.20); schizophrenia, paranoid type (295.30); schizoaffective disorder (295.70); and psychotic disorder not otherwise specified (NOS) (298.9). Patients were diagnosed by a staff psychiatrist upon admission to the facility. Patients with an Axis I diagnosis other than those listed above were not approached to participate in the study.

There were a disproportionate number of male patients because 175 of 200 patients at this facility are male (88%). Also, because the Principal Investigator for this study was the Unit Director for the female unit, this could have presented a conflict of interest. Therefore, due to the small number of female subjects for comparison and generalizability and the potential conflict of interest, females were excluded from this study.

Because the treatment intervention required verbal communication with the participants, and because all staff who administered the intervention are fluent only in English, only patients who read and speak English were approached for participation in the study. Although 9% of the patient population are of ethnicities that do not have English as their primary language, approximately 90% of this patient population read and speak English.

Anticipated length of stay was another criterion for inclusion in the study. Patients admitted to this facility have a variety of commitment statuses that can often predict their length of stay. Some patients are admitted for a brief period of stabilization or evaluation (2-3 weeks) while other patients are admitted for three months or longer. Because the learning of task and interpersonal skills within social roles can be a complex, long-term process, only those patients with anticipated hospitalizations of 30 days or longer were approached to participate in the study.

All patients invited to participate in the study had a Global Assessment of Functioning Scale (GAF) (*DSM-IV-R*, 2000) score of at least 21. The GAF is reported on Axis V of the *DSM-IV-R* multiaxial evaluation and is a report of the psychiatrist's judgement of the individual's overall level of functioning. GAF ratings range from 0 (inadequate information) to 100 (superior functioning in a wide range of activities) in increments of 10. A rating of 1-10 indicates that the patient is in persistent danger of hurting self or others, and a rating of 11-20 indicates that the patient is in some danger of hurting self or others and has a gross impairment in communication. A rating of 21-30 indicates that delusions or hallucinations may considerably influence the patient's behavior, but the patient is no longer a danger to self or others. Therefore, participation in interventions to learn task and interpersonal skills within social role performance could be initiated.

Information regarding inclusion criteria and additional demographic information pertaining to participants' ethnicity, marital status, Axis II diagnosis (*DSM-IV-R*, 2000), psychiatric history, legal status, and level of education was obtained from the participants' hospital records.

A total of 84 patients were admitted to the study with 42 participants each in the experimental and comparison groups. This number reflects a power of .80 to detect a moderate effect size at the .05 level (Cohen, 1988). The statistical power of a test is determined by four factors: the significance criterion, variance in the data, sample size, and effect size (Portnoy & Watkins, 2000). Significance was set at .05. Variance can be reduced by a repeated measures design (Portnoy & Watkins, 2000), and a repeated measures design was used in this study. Effect size was determined to be moderate. Although the Role Development program was considered to be an enhancement of the multidepartmental activity program, the type of treatment involved in the Role Development program and the manner in which it was delivered was substantially different than the existing program, thereby warranting a moderate effect as opposed to a small or large effect. As a result, the sample size was set at 42 in each group for a total sample of 84.

RECRUITMENT PROCEDURES

All participants were asked to sign written informed consent forms describing the research procedures and any anticipated risks. The procedures for the study, the study's anticipated impact on the participant, and any anticipated risks were explained to the participants and repeated back by them to the researcher. The Patient Advocate for the facility co-signed the informed consent form, and remained available to the patients throughout the course of the study to address questions the participant may have been uncomfortable to address with the Principal Investigator. No patient in either group contacted the Patient Advocate during the course of the study. Participants were informed that they were free to withdraw from the research study at any time without prejudicing their access to treatment in any other part of the facility. Although four patients declined to participate in the comparison group and two patients declined to participate in the experimental group, no patients in either group withdrew from the study. Approval for the study was obtained by the institutional review boards at the facility and the university at which the Principal Investigator was completing a doctorate degree.

STAFF PARTICIPANTS IN ROLE DEVELOPMENT TRAINING AND INTERVENTION

The entire rehabilitation department staff (n = 29) participated in the Role Development training. However, because some staff are not in positions involving direct patient care, only 18 staff members implemented Role Development. The facility in which the study occurred has a training policy involving ongoing mandatory training programs for the staff, and the facility viewed the training in Role Development as mandatory training for the rehabilitation staff. This staff training is viewed as one step in the process of continual quality improvement of the rehabilitation program. Therefore, no selection of staff was involved for participation in the study. However, the university's Institutional Review Board requested consent by the rehabilitation staff for program evaluation. Staff consent forms were completed. The researcher conducted focus groups with the rehabilitation staff to gain information and feedback from them. These groups occurred prior to the training in the intervention and once the study was completed. The purpose of these focus groups was (1) to establish staff learning needs prior to training in the intervention entitled Role Development; and (2) to evaluate the effectiveness of the intervention once the study was completed. The Principal Investigator developed questions for each of the focus groups. Approval for this aspect of the study was also obtained by the institutional review boards at the facility and the university at which the Principal Investigator was completing a doctorate degree.

DESIGN–EXPERIMENTAL AND COMPARISON GROUPS

The study used a pretest-posttest design with an experimental group (Role Development program) and a comparison group (multidepartmental activity program) with repeated measures follow-up at four, eight, and 12 weeks (Burns & Grove, 1993; Campbell & Stanley, 1963).

The comparison and experimental groups occurred in a consecutive, as opposed to a concurrent, manner with staff training in Role Development occurring after selection of and data collection for the comparison group, but prior to selection of and data collection for the experimental group. The comparison group participated in the multidepartmental activity program and the experimental group participated in the Role Development program (Schindler, 2002).

Patients who met the criteria for the study and agreed to participate were admitted on an ongoing basis into the comparison group until 42 participants were obtained. Then, the researcher trained the staff participating in the study in the Role Development intervention. Once training was completed, patients who met the criteria for the study and agreed to participate were admitted on an ongoing basis into the experimental group until 42 participants were obtained. Participants remained in the comparison group and the experimental group, respectively, for at least four weeks and up to 12 weeks unless they were discharged from the facility. Patients who were discharged from the facility prior to four weeks were replaced so that the comparison group and experimental group each had 42 patients who completed at least four weeks in the study. The participants who were replaced were excluded from analyses.

To evaluate change over time, participants in both groups were assessed with four instruments (described below) upon admission to the study and at four, eight, and 12 weeks of participation in the study. Those participants involved in the study for less than 12 weeks were assessed for the length of time that they were in the study (i.e., 4 or 8 weeks). Therefore, there were 42 participants for each group at four weeks, but a declining number of participants at eight weeks and a further declining number of participants at 12 weeks.

There were several reasons for conducting the repeated measures. First, it was of interest to measure if there was a difference in the development of skills and roles in shorter versus longer periods of time. Also, because of the inability to control attrition after four weeks and the current reality of short hospital stays, it was important to determine if differences occurred in short periods of time. Lastly, it was important to assess if participants who gain skills and roles continue to improve or are able to sustain these improvements over time.

Comparison Group–Multidepartmental Activity Program

The comparison group participated in the existing multidepartmental activity program (MAP) routinely offered by the facility. The multidepartmental activity program is a non-individualized, therapeutic intervention designed to encourage the productive use of time and socialization in a group setting. Individuals in this program are offered the opportunity to engage in leisure, education, and work-oriented activities and in social interaction with their peers. Intervention is group-oriented and is *not* structured to address the development of individual social roles or the specific skills that are nested in these roles. There is no common link or theoretical foundation among staff using this intervention (Clark et al., 1997).

The multidepartmental activity program occurred on a wing in the facility. This program space is large enough to accommodate all 200 patients. It is comprised of 15 groups occurring simultaneously for each of four 1-hour sessions per day. Monday through Friday patients attend four 1-hour sessions between the hours of 9-11 a.m. and 1:30-3:30 p.m.

The staff involved in the multidepartmental activity program provide occupational therapy, art therapy, and recreation, education, and work-oriented activities. Over 50% of the staff work in recreation. The occupational therapists complete an initial assessment for every patient. Based on the patient's input and performance during the assessment process, and information from the patient's medical record, the occupational therapist assigns the patient to four of the 15 available groups. Professional and paraprofessional rehabilitation staff implement the programs. Over 60% of the staff are paraprofessionals.

The comparison group was comprised of two subgroups: patients participating in the multidepartmental activity program and patients participating in the multidepartmental activity program with individual attention. Because the participants in the experimental group would receive a weekly 15-minute period of individual attention to discuss their development of roles and skills as part of the Role Development program, it was important to assess whether individual attention could be the cause for change. Therefore, it was determined that one-half of the participants in the comparison group would also receive a weekly 15-minute period of individual attention, but this would be in the form of social conversation. Staff were given brief, simple instructions on how to provide individual attention to the participants. Participants assigned odd numbers in the comparison group (1, 3, 5, . . . 41) participated in the regular multidepartmental activity program whereas the participants assigned even numbers (2, 4, 6, . . . 42) participated in the multidepartmental activity program with individual attention. All of these programs are fully described in the operational definitions in Chapter 1.

Experimental Group–Role Development Program

The experimental intervention was a new treatment and an enhancement of the existing multidepartmental activity program. Although the existing program has therapeutic value, because it encourages patients to be involved in activity groups for four hours/day, this intervention is not designed to address a patient's roles or skills, nor is it based on a common theoretical set of guidelines for clinical practice. The Principal Investigator used a theory-based intervention, Role Development, to train the rehabilitation staff. The rehabilitation staff were then able to create theory-based interventions to help each participant develop task and interpersonal skills within meaningful social roles.

A training curriculum (summarized later in this chapter and described fully in Chapter 4) and manual were used to train the staff in Role Development. Once the experimental group began, staff were monitored bi-weekly for fidelity to the intervention via completion of fidelity checklists by the staff and the Principal Investigator. A comprehensive plan to monitor fidelity to the intervention is described in Chapter 4.

INSTRUMENTATION

Four assessments were used in this study: The Role Functioning Scale (Goodman, Sewell, Cooley, & Leavitt, 1993); the Role Checklist (Oakley, 1981); the Task Skills Scale, and the Interpersonal Skills Scale (Mosey, 1986; Rogers, Sciarappa, & Anthony, 1991) (see Table 5). All instruments were used as initial measures of functioning and as repeated posttest measures of functioning for both the experimental and comparison groups. Seven independent raters conducted the initial and repeated measures of functioning. The raters were professional-level staff at the facility with clinical training who work in areas other than the re-

TABLE 5. Instruments

Scale	Authors	Major Factors
Role Functioning Scale (1993)	Goodman, Sewell, Cooley & Leavitt	Working Productivity Independent Living Self-care Independent Social Network Relationships Extended Social Network Relationships
The Role Checklist (1981)	Oakley	Roles
The Task Skills Scale (1986)	Mosey	Task Skills
The Interpersonal Skills Scale (1986; 1991)	Mosey (1986); Rogers, Sciarappa & Anthony (1991)	Interpersonal Skills

habilitation department. Inter-rater reliability was established during the pilot study. It is acknowledged that ratings by independent observers whose reliability is assessed generally yields the most credible results (Durlak, 1998).

The Role Functioning Scale

The Role Functioning Scale (RFS)(Goodman et al., 1993) is a measure of level of functioning of adults in the domains of Working Productivity, Independent Living/Self Care, Immediate Social Network Relationships, and Extended Social Network Relationships. Each domain on the scale is rated from one (a very minimal level of role functioning) to seven (an optimal level of role functioning). Each of the seven points has a behavioral definition. The total of the four scores represents a Global Role Functioning Index with scores ranging from 4 to 28. The authors state that a trained interviewer can complete the scale in a few minutes after a standard interview.

Reliability and validity studies (Goodman et al., 1993) were conducted on the RFS. Four bachelor's or master's level social workers orally administered the instrument to 32 randomly selected women with psychiatric diagnoses, once at the start of the study and again one-year later. The interviewers were blind to the previous data and to the diagnostic category of the participants.

A high level of internal consistency was achieved (Cronbach's alpha = .92). Test-retest reliability for the four scale scores and the Global RFS index ranged from .85 to .92 when administered twice over a one-year interval. Inter-rater reliability correlation ranged from .64 to .82 for the four RFS Scale scores and the Global RFS Index (Goodman et al., 1993).

The validity studies compared women with no psychiatric diagnoses to women with psychiatric diagnoses (N = 112). Criterion group validity tests showed that the well women scored significantly higher (p < .001) than those with psychiatric disorders. For concurrent validity the RFS was compared to two other instruments measuring level of disturbance and self-esteem. It was found that as the Global RFS Index scores increased, there was a corresponding increase in self-esteem (r = .40, p < .001) and a decrease in the severity of psychiatric symptoms (r = .84, p < .001) (Goodman et al., 1993).

A literature search revealed 14 publications documenting the use of the Role Functioning Scale. One of these publications described the development of the scale (McPheeters, 1984). The RFS was originally named the Georgia Role Functioning Scale and was developed as an outcomes measure in the state of Georgia public mental health system. Three publications used the RFS as a model for development of other scales of global functioning (Barker, Barron, McFarland, & Bigelow, 1994; Frazier & Baker-Smith, 1997; Wing et al., 1998). Five publications evaluated or rated the RFS according to specific criteria (Andrews, 1995; Brekke, 1992; Dickerson, 1997; Green & Gracely, 1987; Trauer, 1998). All of these publications favorably reviewed the RFS. Green and Gracely (1987) determined that the RFS attained the highest values for nine of 12 ideal outcome measure criteria developed by a National Institutes of Mental Health (NIMH) task force and ranked second of seven rating scales. In a review of 95 measures of outcome, Andrews (1995) recommended the RFS as one of five measures most suitable for routine outcome measurement. Five publications used the RFS as a measurement tool of psychosocial functioning or global functioning (Brekke & Barrio, 1997; Brekke, Long, Nesbit, & Sobel, 1997; Brekke & Mathiesen, 1995; Brekke, Raine, Ansel, Lencz, & Bird, 1997; Geller, Fisher, McDermeit, & Brown, 1998). Brekke and Mathiesen (1995) used the RFS to measure global functioning of adults diagnosed with schizophrenia living at home with their parents or in noninstitutional settings. Participants living in the noninstitutional settings scored statistically significantly higher on global functioning. Geller, Fisher, McDermeit, and Brown (1998) used the RFS to determine the functional status of patients with multiple inpatient admissions. Those patients with five or more admissions in a single year tended to be lower functioning according to the RFS.

For this study, the Principal Investigator modified the Role Functioning Scale so that it would more accurately reflect the roles available to patients in a maximum-security setting. Three of the domains of the RFS were adapted because the opportunity to develop all roles was limited in this maximum-security setting. The Independent Living/Self Care role was limited to management of eating, sleeping, and hygiene care; household management was eliminated. The category of Immediate Social Network Relationships was limited to friend; spouse and family were eliminated. Extended Social Network Relationships were assessed through participation in hospital-based groups, recreational activities, and church services; neighborhood or community involvement was eliminated. Also, to facilitate a standard approach to the interview for the RFS, a written interview form was developed by the Principal Investigator. This form included an introduction to be read by the rater to the participant and specific questions to assess the roles identified on the

RFS (Interview Form). This form was used at the pretest interview and at each of the posttest interviews. Inter-rater reliability, internal consistency, and test-retest reliability on the RFS were established during the pilot study.

The Role Checklist

The Role Checklist (Barris, Oakley, & Kielhofner, 1988; Oakley, 1981) is a self-report checklist aimed at providing reliable and valid information about an individual's perception of his or her participation in roles and the degree to which each role is valued. The Role Checklist assesses an individual's ability to identify the major roles in his or her life and to indicate the value and importance of the role. Role choices are student, worker, volunteer, caregiver, home maintainer, friend, family member, religious participant, hobbyist/amateur, and participant in organizations. There is also a column labeled "other" in which the individual can write the name of a role that is not listed on the form. The instrument requires approximately 15 minutes to administer and is appropriate for use with an adolescent, adult, or geriatric population with physical or psychiatric disorders. Although the test administrator gives instructions, the Role Checklist has been designed so that the participant can complete the checklist (Oakley, Kielhofner, Barris, & Reichler, 1986).

Content validity, pilot testing, and test-retest reliability were conducted on the instrument. To assess content validity a preliminary list of roles was submitted to graduate students, faculty, and occupational therapists. Feedback from these groups supported the content validity and gave suggestions to further define the roles and avoid sexual stereotyping. Pilot testing was conducted by asking 17 undergraduate students to indicate their perceptions of role occupancy in the past, present and future. To assess test-retest reliability, the Role Checklist was administered to 124 normal volunteers ranging in age from 18 to 79. Kappa and percent agreement scores were calculated for two parts of the instrument. Part One measured perceived incumbency and Part Two measured the degree to which each role is valued. For Part One, kappa for each role ranged from moderate (.41-.60) to substantial (.61-.80), with the majority in the substantial category. Percent agreement for each role ranged from 77%-93%, with an average of 87%. For Part Two, kappa for all roles indicated moderate concordance, and the composite estimate of percent agreement was 79%. The authors concluded that, based on this preliminary study, the Role Checklist is satisfactorily stable with a group of normal adults (Oakley et al., 1986).

A literature search revealed 24 publications documenting the use of the Role Checklist. Nine of these publications addressed the use of the instrument regarding the acquisition of social roles and/or the use of the instrument with individuals diagnosed with mental illness. Oakley, Kielhofner, and Barris (1985) specifically developed the Role Checklist for a study in which they used the instrument, and five other instruments, to assess the adaptive functioning of individuals diagnosed with psychiatric disorders. Data from the six assessments were used to measure the organizational status of 30 individuals. The Role Checklist was adapted for use in the assessment and treatment of an individual diagnosed with multiple personality disorder (Sepiol & Froelich, 1990) and an individual diagnosed with obsessive-compulsive disorder (Bavaro, 1991). Five studies used the Role Checklist as one of several instruments to assess differences in role satisfaction and role functioning among healthy individuals and individuals with physical or psychosocial disabilities (Barris, Dickie, & Baron, 1988; Ebb, Coster, & Duncombe, 1989; Oakley & Dickerson, 1995; Smyntek, Barris, & Kielhofner, 1985) and juvenile delinquency (Lededer, Kielhofner, & Watts, 1985). All of these studies found discrepancies in the number of roles and the value given to roles between the healthy and disabled populations. The Role Checklist was also used to assess role preferences and life satisfaction in a healthy adult population (Branholm & Fugl-Meyer, 1992).

For this study, the Principal Investigator modified the Role Checklist to better address the needs of the participants. The roles of home maintainer and hobbyist/amateur were eliminated, and the role of participant in organizations was changed to group member. Also, instead of evaluating the degree of value a participant placed on a role, this was changed to assess the level of satisfaction a participant attributed to past performance of the role (i.e., not satisfied, somewhat satisfied, or very satisfied in past performance of the role). All roles in the Role Checklist were included in the assessment of the patient's past and future participation in roles and level of satisfaction with roles. However, because this study was conducted in a maximum-security setting, participants did not have the opportunity to develop all roles listed in the Role Checklist. Therefore, the roles the patient could choose to develop during the study were limited to the roles of student, worker, friend, and group member. Additionally, because the Role Checklist was not designed for the purpose of pretest-posttest evaluation, a written form was developed by the Principal Investigator to record the participant's perception of progress in developing roles. This form (Follow-up Questions to the Role Checklist) has specific questions for the rater to ask the participant concerning roles he identified he wanted to develop at the time of the pretest. This instrument was assessed for feasibility during the pilot study.

Task Skills Scale and Interpersonal Skills Scale

The Task Skills Scale and the Interpersonal Skills Scale were developed by the Principal Investigator and were derived primarily from the continuums and behaviors of function and dysfunction in the Role Acquisition frame of reference (Mosey, 1986, pp. 453-454) and from the Interpersonal Skills Scale (Rogers, Sciarappa, & Anthony, 1991, p. 65). Modifications were made to better meet the needs of the participants in this study. These scales were used to assess the eight identified task skills and the eight identified interpersonal skills that are addressed in Role Development. It was estimated that a trained interviewer would be able to complete this instrument in 15 minutes after observing participants involved in tasks and social interactions for one-half hour.

Because the Task Skills Scale and Interpersonal Skills Scale were developed by the Principal Investigator for use in this study, there is no literature on their prior use. However, there is literature on the Interpersonal Skills Scale developed by Rogers, Sciarappa, and Anthony (1991). These authors developed an Interpersonal Skills Scale and a Work Adjustment Scale as instruments to conduct situational assessments. The Interpersonal Skills Scale contains 14 items and the Work Adjustment Scale contains 21 items. Reliability and validity were conducted with 50 subjects diagnosed with schizophrenic disorders. Inter-rater reliability for the Interpersonal Skills Scale was $r = .75$ ($p < .001$), coefficient alpha was .97, and test-retest reliability was .76 ($p < .001$, $N = 41$, rater #1) and .72 ($p < .001$, $N = 43$, rater #2). Discriminant analyses were performed to determine predictive validity, and these functions were able to correctly predict employment status for 54% to 87% of subjects. Concurrent validity was analyzed using the Griffith's Work Behavior Scale. Results suggested adequate correlations ($r = .49$, $p < .01$, $N = 24$) with the first rater on the Interpersonal Skills Scale but were not statistically significant with the second rater (.46, $p > .01$, $N = 24$).

Inter-rater reliability, test-retest reliability, and internal consistency for the Task Skills Scale and the Interpersonal Skills Scale were established during the pilot study.

PILOT STUDY

A pilot study was conducted to assess potential problems or concerns with the actual study and to establish inter-rater reliability, internal consistency, and test-retest reliability on three scales: (1) Role Functioning Scale (Goodman, Sewell, Cooley, & Leavitt, 1993); (2) Task Skills Scale; and (3) Interpersonal Skills Scale (Mosey, 1986; Rogers, Sciarappa, & Anthony, 1991). The pilot study also examined the feasibility of using the Role Checklist (Oakley, 1981).

Four raters were recruited for the reliability studies. All raters are staff at the facility who have clinical backgrounds, although they are currently working in administrative or staff training positions. Training in the administration of the scales was conducted. A schedule was developed in which each staff rater was paired with every other rater (e.g., R1/R2, R1/R3, R1/R4, R2/R3, etc.). Each pair was scheduled to observe, interview and rate five patients.

Once the pilot study was underway, it became apparent that: (1) additional training was needed for a consistent approach among the raters; (2) a more specific interview was needed to obtain information to adequately complete the Role Functioning Scale; and (3) language revisions were needed to rate the Task Skills Scale and the Interpersonal Skills Scale. Drafts of the interview and rating scale were developed and evaluated. When the Principal Investigator and staff raters concluded that the revised tools addressed the problems, training followed. Once the training was complete, the pilot study was reinitiated.

A total of 12 patients were observed and interviewed by four raters, and the rating scales were completed. The age of the patients ranged from 18-49; the mean age was 37 years with a standard deviation of 8.4. Eight of the patients were Caucasian (66%) and four of the patients were African American (33%). Eleven of the patients were never married (92%) and one patient was divorced (8%). Length of stay varied from less than one month to greater than one year; the mean was 2-3 months with a standard deviation of 2.1.

Inter-rater reliability and internal consistency were obtained for all three scales (see Table 6).

Alpha Coefficients

Alpha coefficients were conducted on three scales. Alpha coefficient for the Role Functioning Scale (N = 16) was .98. Alpha coefficient for the Task Skills Scale was .99 (N = 32); for the Interpersonal Skills Scale

TABLE 6. Alpha Coefficients, Inter-rater Reliability, and Test-Retest Reliability: Pilot Study N = 12

Scale	Alpha Coefficient	Inter-rater Reliability	Test-Retest Reliability
Role Functioning	.98	.84-.97	.81-.92
Interpersonal Skills	.99	.70-.88	.82-1.0
Task Skills Scale	.99	.81-.93	.81-.93

it was .99 (N = 32). To assess inter-rater reliability, bivariate correlations were conducted on every item in every scale for all four raters (Role Functioning Scale–four items; Task Skills Scale–eight items; Interpersonal Skills Scale–eight items) (see Table 6).

Inter-rater Reliability of Three Scales

The Role Functioning Scale had correlations ranging from .84-.97: independent living/self-care (.84); working productivity (.84); immediate social network relationships (.87); and extended social network relationships (.97).

The Interpersonal Skills Scale had correlations ranging from .70-.88: interacts comfortably with peers (.70); interacts comfortably with staff (.73); communicates accurately and expresses self clearly (.75); controls impulsive, offensive, and/or annoying behavior (.75); keeps all statements appropriate to context (.79); ability to initiate, respond to, and sustain verbal interactions (.80); uses appropriate non-verbal behavior and tone of voice (.83); cooperates as a member of a group (.88).

The Task Skills Scale had correlations ranging from .81-.93: tolerates frustration (.81); ability to organize task in a logical manner (.86); willingness to engage in doing tasks (.87); rate of performance (.88); attention to detail (.88); ability to follow directions (.90); ability to maintain concentration on task (.90); and physical capacity (.93).

All staff raters and the Principal Investigator concluded that the Role Checklist was a viable tool with valuable information. Patients commented that this tool focused on their needs as individuals. One minor revision was made (i.e., religious participant was excluded as a role that could be developed at the facility during the course of the study), but the checklist otherwise remained intact.

Once inter-rater reliability and internal consistency were established, a pilot study to determine test-retest reliability was conducted.

A total of 12 patients were observed and interviewed by three raters, and the rating scales were completed. These patients were observed and interviewed on two consecutive Tuesday afternoons, at the same time of day, in the same rehabilitation group (i.e., workshop), and by the same raters. Demographics and correlations described pertain to 11 patients because one of the patients severely decompensated in the span of one week. The age of the patients ranged from 26-54; the mean age was 41 years with a standard deviation of 8.9. Nine of the patients were Caucasian (82%) and two of the patients were African American (18%). Ten of the patients were never married (91%) and one patient was widowed (9%). Length of stay varied from less than one month to greater than one year; the mean was 2-3 months with a standard deviation of 1.7. Test-retest reliability was obtained for the Role Functioning Scale, the Task Skills Scale and the Interpersonal Skills Scale (see Table 6).

To assess test-retest reliability, bivariate correlations were conducted on every item in every scale (Role Functioning Scale–four items; Task Skills Scale–eight items; Interpersonal Skills Scale–eight items).

The Role Functioning Scale had correlations ranging from .81-.92: independent living/self-care (.81); working productivity (.92); immediate social network relationships (.86); and extended social network relationships (.90).

The Interpersonal Skills Scale had correlations ranging from .82-1.0: interacts comfortably with peers (.82); interacts comfortably with staff (.84); communicates accurately and expresses self clearly (.89); controls impulsive, offensive, and/or annoying behavior (.90); keeps all statements appropriate to context (.85); ability to initiate, respond to, and sustain verbal interactions (1.0); uses appropriate non-verbal behavior and tone of voice (.86); cooperates as a member of a group (.89).

The Task Skills Scale had correlations ranging from .81-.93: tolerates frustration (.93); ability to organize task in a logical manner (.81); willingness to engage in doing tasks (.87); rate of performance (.82); attention to detail (.87); ability to follow directions (.82); ability to maintain concentration on task (.93); and physical capacity (.93).

Procedure

The study was completed over the course of 13 months. A total of 84 patients participated in the study that was conducted at a maximum-security state forensic facility. Patients were invited to participate as they were admitted to the facility and met the criteria for inclusion in the study. A timeline indicating the course of events in the study is outlined in Table 7.

TABLE 7. Timeline and Sequence of Activity for the Research Study

Date	Research Activity
Months 1-5	42 participants enrolled in and completed Comparison Group
Month 6	PI Interviewed Patient Participants who completed 12 weeks in Comparison Group
Months 6-10	PI conducted Rehabilitation Staff Training
Months 7-12	42 participants enrolled in and completed Experimental Group
Month 13	PI Interviewed Patient Participants who completed 12 weeks in Experimental Group

Procedure for Pretest and Posttest Evaluations

Immediately after a participant agreed to participate in the study and sign the written consent form, the participant was assigned to a rater. All raters involved in the study achieved inter-rater reliability prior to conducting an evaluation. Within three days of the assignment, the rater went to the rehabilitation wing to conduct the pretest evaluation. The rater observed the participant in a group setting and conducted an individual, private interview with the client. The observation was scheduled for 30 minutes and the interview took an average of 20 to 30 minutes to complete. To conduct the observation the rater sat in an inconspicuous location in the group area and observed the client. Then, the rater and the participant moved to the Interview Room to conduct the interview required to complete the Role Functioning Scale and the Role Checklist. The rater used the Interview Questions developed by the Principal Investigator to conduct the interview and also completed the Role Checklist with the participant during this time.

The rater was instructed to complete the Task Skills Scale, Interpersonal Skills Scale and the Role Functioning Scale immediately after conducting the observation and interview and return the folder with these scales to the Principal Investigator. The patient participant and rater were assigned separate identification numbers. The group and location in which the participant was observed was recorded so that the participant could be observed in the same group and location for each of the posttests.

The same procedure was followed for each of the posttests with the exception of the rater using the Follow-up Questions to the Role Checklist in place of the Role Checklist.

Recruitment and Participation of Comparison Group

Over the course of 11 weeks, 42 participants were enrolled in the comparison group. Forty-seven participants were recruited for the study. Four participants declined to participate. One participant was discharged from the facility prior to the first posttest, and this participant was subsequently replaced. Forty-two participants completed one posttest (4 weeks in the study), 20 participants completed two posttests (8 weeks in the study) and 17 participants completed three posttests (12 weeks in the study) (see Table 8). All of the patients participated in the multidepartmental activity program throughout their duration in the study. Additionally, 21 participants (one-half of the sample and every other participant enrolled in the comparison group) received up to 15 minutes of individual attention per week from all of their group leaders.

Upon completion of the comparison group, all participants who completed 12 weeks in the comparison group (N = 17) were interviewed regarding their thoughts and perceptions about their participation in the program.

Staff Training

Twenty-nine rehabilitation staff were trained over 10 weeks for a total of 15.5 hours of training. Although 29 staff were trained, not all staff implemented the training. Five of the staff were in supervisory positions and do not carry a patient caseload, two were students who had left the facility, and two staff did not have caseloads for administrative reasons. Therefore, 20 staff had the potential to implement the training. Eighteen staff actually had patients enrolled in the study (Occupational Therapy [4], Art Therapy [1], Vocational Rehabilitation [1], Education [2], Recreation [10]). (See Table 9.)

TABLE 8. Number of Patient Participants in the Research Study

Group	# Declined participation	# Replaced	Posttest 1 (4 weeks)	Posttest 2 (8 weeks)	Posttest 3 (12 weeks)
			n = 42		
Comparison	4	1	42	20	17
			n = 42		
Experimental	2	3	42	17	11

TABLE 9. Staff Implementing Role Development

Staff: Title:	Rehab Director	Rehab Supervisor	OT/AT Staff	Recreation Staff	Voc Rehab/ Education Staff	Total
Staff: n =	0	0	5	10	3	18

A curriculum was developed for the training. The rehabilitation staff were educated through a variety of techniques. A staff training manual based on the set of guidelines for practice (see Chapters 3 and 4) was developed and each staff member participating in the training received a copy of the manual. This served as the primary resource for the training and for the staff to use as a reference to develop and monitor the implementation of Role Development with their patients enrolled in the experimental group. Formal group training was conducted for 1-2 hours per week for 10 weeks for a total of 15.5 hours and included didactic instruction, small work-group instruction, and homework assignments. During formal training, staff had multiple opportunities to practice the assessment of skills and roles and develop treatment plans prior to the implementation of the study. Formal training concluded with each staff member demonstrating integration and application of Role Development through successful completion of a case-study assignment. Individual training followed formal training. In the individual training, the Principal Investigator observed each staff member as he/she conducted a group session. Upon completion of the observation, the Principal Investigator and the staff member brainstormed appropriate methods to implement Role Development with patients in his/her group.

Recruitment and Participation of the Experimental Group

Once the training was completed, the Principal Investigator began to recruit patients for the experimental phase of the study. Over the course of 14 weeks (recruitment was interrupted during the holiday season), 42 participants were enrolled in the experimental group. Forty-seven participants were recruited for the study. Two participants declined to participate. Three participants were discharged from the facility prior to the first posttest; these participants were replaced. Forty-two participants completed one posttest (4 weeks in the study), 17 participants completed two posttests (8 weeks in the study) and 11 participants completed three posttests (12 weeks in the study) (see Table 7). These patients participated in the Role Development program throughout their duration in the study.

Upon completion of the experimental group, all participants who completed 12 weeks in the experimental group (N = 11) were interviewed regarding their thoughts and perceptions about their participation in the study.

Staff Fidelity to Role Development

To monitor fidelity to Role Development during the implementation of the experimental aspect of the study, several measures were implemented. Staff were required to complete an initial treatment plan and a weekly progress report on each of their patients involved in the study. Forms were created to complete this documentation and were part of the staff training manual. Compliance with completion of these forms was required, recorded, and shared with the staff member's supervisor. A weekly one-hour meeting was held with all staff involved in the Role Development program to discuss progress or lack of progress for each participant involved in the study. Attendance was mandatory and recorded. At least once every two weeks the Principal Investigator observed each staff member involved in the Role Development program with one of his/her patients. Upon completion of this observation, both the Principal Investigator and the staff member completed a Fidelity Checklist.

DATA ANALYSIS

The data were analyzed using the *Statistical Package of Social Sciences (SPSS)* for Windows, versions 6.1 and 10.0 (Norusis, no date provided). The statistical significance level of .05 was selected for data analysis (Cohen, 1988).

Data analysis was approached in the following manner. For tests in which there are equivalent parametric and nonparametric tests (e.g., *t*-test–Mann-Whitney; Pearson-Product Moment Correlation–Spearman-rho), both tests were conducted. In these cases, the parametric and nonparametric equivalent tests consistently produced the same type of findings (i.e., statistically significant or non-significant). Because the instruments used in the study more closely represent ordinal rather than interval level data, the Principal Investigator chose to report the more conservative nonparametric findings. However, in cases where the test was important to conduct, but there is no nonparametric equivalent (e.g., ANCOVA,

MANCOVA, repeated measures ANOVA), these parametric findings are reported.

Data analysis began with descriptive statistics for the sample. Tests were conducted to determine pretest differences between the comparison and experimental groups on all of the demographic variables and on the Role Functioning Scale, Task Skills Scale, and Interpersonal Skills Scale. There were no pretest differences in the Role Functioning Scale, but pretest differences did exist in the Task Skills Scale and the Interpersonal Skills Scale. Additional analyses were conducted to determine the nature of the pretest differences. As there were no pretest differences in the Role Functioning Scale, further tests were conducted to measure within-group and between-group differences. Because there were pretest differences in the Task Skills Scale and the Interpersonal Skills Scale, an ANCOVA and within-group tests were conducted. The ANCOVA is a useful test in a pretest-posttest design if differences occur in groups on the pretest (Burns & Grove, 1993), and within-group tests were helpful to understand change over time. Repeated Measures ANOVA was conducted on each of the three scales to measure differences between the experimental and comparison groups over three periods of time (Green, Salkind, & Akey, 2000). Because the research design for this study included attrition after completion of the first posttest (i.e., 4 weeks) for both the comparison and experimental groups, data at eight and 12 weeks of the study were analyzed with decreasing N's. Finally, a MANCOVA was conducted to determine if there were statistically significant mean differences among the comparison and experimental groups after adjusting the dependent variable (a linear combination of the three dependent variables–Task Skills Scale [TSS], Interpersonal Skills Scale [ISS] and the Role Functioning Scale [RFS]: Mertler & Vannatta, 2002).

Because the Role Checklist is a self-report measure, summary statistics were conducted for the comparison and experimental groups. Comparisons were made between groups on the types of roles participants selected as roles to develop.

Two other types of data were collected and analyzed to present a more comprehensive analysis of the findings. Descriptive data on the staff implementing Role Development were collected and analyzed to provide information on the characteristics of staff involved. Bivariate correlation coefficients were conducted on variables indicative of staff fidelity to the Role Development intervention. Also, qualitative interviews were conducted to understand both staff and patient perceptions regarding change. Patients who participated for the entire 12-week period of the comparison or experimental group were interviewed at the conclusion of each phase of the study. The findings are included as anecdotal information. Also, staff focus groups were conducted prior to staff training and at the conclusion of the study. The staff focus groups were recorded and transcribed. Trends were identified and themes were developed and analyzed.

STAFF FOCUS GROUPS

Prior to staff training, the Principal Investigator met with 24 rehabilitation staff in pre-training focus groups, and after the completion of the study, the Principal Investigator met with 22 rehabilitation staff in post-study focus groups. Separate focus groups included the following participants: Rehabilitation Director (N = 1); Rehabilitation Supervisors (N = 4); and Rehabilitation Staff (N = 9) in three separate groups–occupational therapy/art therapy (N = 7 pre-training; N = 5 post-study), recreation (N = 9), vocational rehabilitation/education (N = 3) (see Table 10). Five questions were addressed in the pre-training focus group, and seven questions were addressed in the post-study focus group. The focus groups are described in detail in Chapter 9.

TABLE 10. Staff Participating in Pretest and Posttest Focus Groups

Staff	Rehab Director	Rehab Supervisor	OT/AT Staff	Recreation Staff	Voc Rehab/ Education Staff	Total
Staff: n =	1	4	7/5*	9	3	24/22**

*= 7 in Pre-training Focus Group; 5 in Post-study Focus Group
**= 24 in Pre-training Focus Group; 22 in Post-study Focus Group

Chapter 6

Evaluating the Effectiveness of Role Development: Quantitative Data

This study consisted of a repeated measures design in which 42 participants in an experimental group (Role Development program) and a comparison group (multidepartmental activity program) (N = 84) were measured on four dependent variables (Task Skills Scale, Interpersonal Skills Scale, Role Functioning Scale, and the Role Checklist) at pretest and three posttests.

This chapter begins with demographic data on the study sample followed by results of the pretests. Then, the findings are presented by addressing each of the four research hypotheses. The chapter finishes with a conclusion.

THE PATIENT PARTICIPANTS

The demographic data were organized into five categorical (ethnicity, marital status, legal status, Axis I diagnosis, Axis II Diagnosis) (see Table 11) and four continuous (age, education, psychiatric history, length of stay) variables (see Table 12).

A total of 84 men participated in the study. The age of the participants ranged from 18 to 55 (mean age 33.5). The majority of the participants were African American (67.9%) followed by Caucasian (22.6%), Hispanic (8.3%) and Asian (1.2%). The participants were relatively under-

[Haworth co-indexing entry note]: "Evaluating the Effectiveness of Role Development: Quantitative Data." Schindler, Victoria P. Co-published simultaneously in *Occupational Therapy in Mental Health* (The Haworth Press, Inc.) Vol. 20, No. 3/4, 2004, pp. 79-104; and: *Occupational Therapy in Forensic Psychiatry: Role Development and Schizophrenia* (Victoria P. Schindler) The Haworth Press, Inc., 2004, pp. 79-104. Single or multiple copies of this article are available for a fee from The Haworth Document Delivery Service [1-800-HAWORTH, 9:00 a.m. - 5:00 p.m. (EST). E-mail address: docdelivery@haworthpress.com].

http://www.haworthpress.com/web/OTMH
Digital Object Identifier: 10.1300/J004v20n03_06

TABLE 11. Demographic Data for Total Participants: Categorical Variables (n = 84)

Categorical Variable	Total Group		Comparison		Experimental	
	N	%	N	%	N	%
Ethnicity						
Asian	1	1.2	1	2.4	0	0.0
Hispanic	7	8.3	4	9.5	3	7.1
Caucasian	19	22.6	7	16.7	12	28.6
African American	57	67.9	30	71.4	27	64.3
Marital Status						
Married	1	1.2	0	0.0	1	1.2
Divorced	9	10.7	3	7.1	6	14.3
Never Married	74	88.1	39	92.9	35	83.3
Legal Status						
Prison	11	13.1	6	14.3	5	11.9
Max Out	15	18.0	7	16.7	8	19.0
State Hospital	23	27.0	14	33.3	10	23.8
Jail	35	42.0	15	35.7	19	45.2
Axis I Diagnosis						
SCZ, Disorganized	1	1.2	1	2.4	0	0.0
SCZ, Residual	6	7.1	1	2.4	5	11.9
Psychotic Disorder	7	8.3	0	0.0	7	16.7
SCZ, Undifferen.	8	9.5	4	9.5	4	9.5
SCZ, Paranoid	24	28.6	15	35.7	9	21.4
Schizoaffective	38	45.2	21	50.0	17	40.5
Axis II Diagnosis						
Paranoid PD	1	1.2	1	2.4	0	0.0
Personality Dis	1	1.2	1	2.4	0	0.0
Borderline PD	7	8.3	4	9.5	3	7.1
Antisocial PD	23	27.4	9	21.4	14	33.3
None listed	53	62.0	27	64.3	25	59.5

educated. Over 75% of the participants had some high school or less. Thirteen participants had an elementary education (15.5%); 11 participants were classified as special education (13.1%); and 41 participants had some high school (49%).

Only 17 participants had a high school diploma (20.2%); some college (1.2%); or a college degree (1.2%). Over three-quarters of the par-

TABLE 12. Demographic Data for the Participants: Continuous Variables
(n = 84)

Categorical Variable	Total Group		Comparison		Experimental	
	N	%	N	%	N	%
Age						
<20	6	7.1	1	2.4	5	11.9
<30	24	28.6	13	30.9	11	26.2
<40	34	40.5	19	45.3	15	35.7
<50	17	20.2	8	19.0	9	21.4
<55	3	3.6	1	2.4	2	4.8
Education						
Elementary	13	15.5	3	7.1	10	23.8
Special Education	11	13.1	7	16.7	4	9.5
Some High School	41	49.0	21	50.0	20	47.6
High School Diploma	17	20.2	9	21.4	8	19.0
Some College	1	1.2	1	2.4	0	0.0
College Degree	1	1.2	1	2.4	0	0.0
Psychiatric History						
First Contact	9	10.7	1	2.4	8	19.0
6 months – 1 year	1	1.2	1	2.4	0	0.0
1-5 years	20	23.8	11	26.2	9	21.4
5-10 years	18	21.4	11	26.2	7	16.7
Greater than 10 years	34	40.5	16	38.1	18	42.9
Unknown	2	2.4	2	2.4	0	0.0
Length of Stay						
1-2 months	47	56.0	22	52.4	25	59.5
2-3 months	10	12.0	3	7.1	6	14.3
3-6 months	27	32.0	17	40.5	11	26.2

ticipants were never married (88.1%). One participant was married (1.2%) and nine participants (10.7%) were divorced. Although psychiatric history ranged from first psychiatric contact to greater than 10 years, the majority of participants had a psychiatric history of at least five years. Psychiatric history was recorded as first psychiatric contact (10.7%); six months to one year (1.2%); one to five years (23.8%); five to 10 years (21.4%); greater than 10 years (40.5%); and unknown (2.4%). Legal status was recorded according to the levels of legal commitment established at the facility. They include: admitted from/returning to prison (13.1%); maxed out of prison/to be discharged to a state psychiatric hospital (18%); admitted from a state psychiatric hospital/returning to a state psychiatric hospital (27%); admitted from a county jail/returning to a county jail or a state psychiatric hospital (42%).

Six Axis I diagnoses within the Schizophrenic Disorders described in *DSM-IV-R* (2000) were represented: schizophrenia, disorganized (1.2%); schizophrenia, residual (7.1%); psychotic disorder, NOS (8.3%); schizophrenia, undifferentiated (9.5%); schizophrenia, paranoid (28.6%); schizoaffective disorder (45.2%) (see Table 11).

Four Axis II diagnoses within the Personality Disorders described in *DSM-IV-R* (2000) were represented, although the majority of participants had no Axis II diagnosis. The Axis II diagnoses included: paranoid personality disorder (1.2%); personality disorder, NOS (1.2%); borderline personality disorder (8.3%); antisocial personality disorder (27.4 %); no personality disorder listed (62%) (see Table 11).

Length of stay varied from less than one month to three to six months. However, those participants discharged from the facility prior to one month were eliminated from the study and replaced. Those clients remaining three to six months were included for the entire 12 weeks of the study. Length of stay was recorded as 1-2 months (56%); 2-3 months (12%); 3-6 months (32%) (see Table 12).

RESULTS OF PRETESTS

The Chi-square test was used to assess pretest differences on the categorical variables (ethnicity, marital status, legal status, Axis I diagnosis, Axis II diagnosis). The Mann-Whitney U test was used to assess pretest differences on the continuous variables (education, psychiatric history, and length of stay). Because these variables were organized into ranks, the nonparametric test was used. A t-test was used to compare pretest differences on age. There were no statistically significant differences between the groups in each of the nine descriptive variables (age, p = .59; ethnicity, p = .14; marital status, p = .51; education p = .16; psychiatric history, p = .32; legal status, p = .39; Axis I diagnosis, p = .80; Axis II diagnosis, p = .58 and length of stay, p = .34).

The Mann-Whitney U test was used to assess pretest differences in the Role Functioning Scale, Task Skills Scale, and the Interpersonal Skills Scale. Because all of these scales collected ordinal-level data, this nonparametric test was used. There was no pretest difference in the

Role Functioning Scale ($Z = -.1212$; $p = .90$). However, there were statistically significant pretest differences in the Task Skills Scale (TSS) ($Z = -3.0553$; $p = .002$) and the Interpersonal Skills Scale (ISS) ($Z = -2.5309$; $p = .01$). The data were carefully examined and analyzed to determine the nature of the pretest differences on these two scales. Pretest scores for the eight items on each scale were plotted for the Task Skills Scale and Interpersonal Skills Scale for both the comparison and experimental groups. The Task Skills Scale showed the greatest amount of pretest difference.

An analysis of pretest differences between the comparison and experimental groups on the Task Skills Scale and the Interpersonal Skills Scale indicated that there was a subgroup within each group that may have caused the differences.

Comparison Group

For the comparison group a subgroup of patients scored higher on the pretest with a subsequent decrease on posttest 1. The demographic data and the raters completing the scales on this subgroup of 10 participants were examined for similarities. The only variable showing some similarity was the demographic variable of psychiatric history. Seven of these 10 clients (70%) had a psychiatric history of greater than 10 years (as compared to 38% of the total comparison group and 40% of the total sample). Three of these 10 clients (30%) had a psychiatric history of five to 10 years (as compared to 26% of the total comparison group and 21% of the total sample). Therefore, all of these clients had a psychiatric history of greater than five years. Perhaps these clients presented with greater skills shortly after admission (pretest) but became less involved in the multidepartmental activity program as their hospital stay progressed. Subsequent patient interviews support that these patients may have lost interest in the program.

Experimental Group

For the experimental group a subgroup of patients scored lower than the total experimental group on the pretest with a subsequent increase on posttest 1. The demographic data and the raters completing the scales on this subgroup of 13 participants were also examined for similarities. Three variables (Axis II diagnosis, psychiatric history and education) showed some similarity. Seven of the 13 participants (54%) had a psychiatric history of greater than 10 years (as compared to 38% of the comparison group and 40% of the total sample). Six of the 13 subgroup participants (46%) had an Axis II diagnosis of Antisocial Personality Disorder (as compared to 33% of the experimental group and 27% of the total sample). Five of the 13 participants (46%) had an education level of elementary school (as compared to 24% of the experimental group and 15% of the total sample). Perhaps the combination of factors (psychiatric history of greater than 10 years, Axis II diagnosis of Antisocial Personality Disorder and elementary school education) had an influence on low pretest scores. Subsequent quantitative and qualitative findings support the improved scores for this group.

ANALYSIS OF COVARIANCE

The first two research hypotheses addressed the Task Skills Scale and the Interpersonal Skills Scale and were written as follows: (1) Adults diagnosed with schizophrenic disorders will demonstrate greater improvement in task skills (as evidenced by a statistically significant improvement in scores on the Task Skills Scale) when involved in individualized intervention based on Role Development in comparison to participation in a multidepartmental activity program; and (2) Adults diagnosed with schizophrenic disorders demonstrate greater improvement in interpersonal skills (as evidenced by a statistically significant improvement in scores on the Interpersonal Skills Scale) when involved in individualized intervention based on Role Development in comparison to participation in a multidepartmental activity program.

A test to address the first two hypotheses is an analysis of covariance (ANCOVA). An ANCOVA was conducted with the Task Skills Scale and the Interpersonal Skills Scale because these scales had differences on the pretests. An analysis of covariance can be a useful approach to analysis in pretest-posttest designs in which differences occur in groups on the pretest. In this case, an ANCOVA maximizes the capacity to detect differences by incorporating the covariates (Burns & Grove, 1993). Tests of between-subject effects were completed with the comparison and experimental groups serving as the between-subjects factors. The ANCOVA was run twice and the results are summarized in Table 13. First, the Task Skills Scale pretest scores were used as the covariate. The results showed a statistically significant difference ($p = .000$). In the second test, the Interpersonal Skills Scale pretest scores were used as the covariate. The results showed a statistically significant difference ($p = .000$).

TABLE 13. Analysis of Covariance: Tests of Between-Subjects Effects

Dependent variable: Task Skills Scale Posttest 1

Source	Type III Sum of Squares	Df	Mean Square	F	p
Corrected Model	879.526	2	439.763	13.745	.000
TSSPRE	750.764	1	750.764	23.466	.000
Type	381.022	1	381.022	11.909	.001
Error (within)	2591.474	81	31.994	-	-

Dependent variable: Interpersonal Skills Scale Posttest 1

Source	Type III Sum of Squares	Df	Mean Square	F	P
Corrected Model	906.844	2	453.422	21.577	.000
ISSPRE	801.654	1	801.654	38.149	.000
Type	309.330	1	309.330	14.720	.000
Error (within)	1702.108	81	21.014	-	-

The findings of the ANCOVA in regards to the first two hypotheses indicated that participants in the experimental group demonstrated statistically significant differences in their task skills and interpersonal skills when compared to the participants in the comparison group.

TASK SKILLS SCALE

The first research hypothesis addressed the Task Skills Scale. To supplement findings from the ANCOVA regarding this hypothesis, within-group tests were conducted. Pretest differences between the comparison and experimental groups on the Task Skills Scale limited data analysis to within-group tests. Also, within-group tests were used to determine the degree of change at each of the posttests. Mean, standard deviation and difference scores from pretest to posttest 1 were calculated for the comparison and experimental groups. Because ordinal data were collected, the Wilcoxon Matched-Pairs Signed-Ranks Test was used to make within-group comparisons. The mean, z, and p scores for the Task Skills Scale are summarized in Table 14. Comparison of scores from pretest to posttest 1 (n = 42, p = .44), posttest 1 to posttest 2 (n = 20, p = .44), and posttest 2 to posttest 3 (n = 17, p = .66) for the com-

TABLE 14. Task Skills Scale: Comparison of Posttest Findings Within Comparison and Experimental Groups

	Post 1 (4 weeks)			Post 2 (8 weeks)			Post 3 (12 weeks)		
	N	M	z	p	N	M	Z	P	N	M	z	p
C	42	−.54	−0.76	.446	20	+0.75	−0.76	.447	17	+0.47	−0.49	.622
E	42	+6.16	−5.40	.000	17	+2.90	−2.80	.005	11	+1.50	−1.40	.173

M = mean change scores

parison group all revealed no statistically significant findings. However, comparison of scores for the experimental group for pretest to posttest 1 (n = 42, p = .000), posttest 1 to posttest 2 (n = 17, p = .005), and posttest 2 to posttest 3 (n = 11, p = .17) revealed statistically significant findings for the four week and eight week posttest.

These findings indicate that the participants in the Role Development program demonstrated greater improvement in task skills than participants involved in the multidepartmental activity program at four and eight weeks of treatment. Although the findings at 12 weeks of treatment for the experimental group are not statistically significant (p = .173), mean scores increased from eight weeks of treatment. This may indicate that although the participants in the experimental group did not demonstrate statistically significant improvement at week 12, they were able to maintain or slightly increase their level of task skills over their initial scores. Mean scores for the comparison group decreased from pretest scores at four weeks of treatment indicating a decline in task skills from the pretest. Although mean scores increased slightly at eight and 12 weeks of treatment, none of the increases qualify as statistically significant improvement in task skills for this group.

INTERPERSONAL SKILLS SCALE

The second research hypothesis addressed the Interpersonal Skills Scale. As with the Task Skills Scale, because there were pretest differences between the comparison and experimental groups on the Interpersonal Skills Scale, data analysis was limited to within-group tests. Mean, standard deviation and difference scores from pretest to posttest 1 were calculated for the comparison and experimental groups. Because ordinal data were collected, the Wilcoxon Matched-Pairs Signed-Ranks Test was used to make within-group comparisons. The z scores and p scores for the Interpersonal Skills Scale are summarized in Table 15. Comparison of scores from pretest to posttest 1 (n = 42, p = .52), posttest 1 to posttest 2 (n = 20, p = .42), and posttest 2 to posttest 3 (n = 17, p = .82) for the comparison group all revealed no statistically significant findings. However, comparison of scores for the experimental group for pretest to posttest 1 (n = 42, p = .000), posttest 1 to posttest 2 (n = 17, p = .07), and posttest 2 to posttest 3 (n = 11, p = .34) revealed statistically significant findings for the four week posttest.

Findings from these tests indicate that the participants in the Role Development program demonstrated greater improvement in interpersonal skills than participants involved in the multidepartmental activity program at four weeks of treatment. Although the findings at eight (p = .079) and 12 weeks (p = .344) of treatment for the experimental group are not statistically significant, the mean scores show continuing improvement at both of these pretests. This may indicate that the participants in the experimental group were able to greatly improve their interpersonal skills in the first four weeks of treatment and maintain their level of interpersonal skills. The mean scores for the participants in the comparison group demonstrate a slight increase at each of the posttests indicating that these participants may have shown slight improvement in interpersonal skills.

ROLE FUNCTIONING SCALE

The third research hypothesis specifically addressed the Role Functioning Scale and the Role Checklist and was written as follows: Adults diagnosed with schizophrenic disorders develop more social roles (as evidenced by a statistically significant improvement in scores on the Role Functioning Scale and a greater number of roles on the Role Checklist) when involved in individualized intervention based on Role Development in comparison to participation in a multidepartmental activity program. The findings of the Role Functioning Scale will be presented first.

TABLE 15. Interpersonal Skills Scale: Comparison of Posttest Findings Within Comparison and Experimental Groups

	Post 1 (4 weeks)				Post 2 (8 weeks)				Post 3 (12 weeks)			
	N	M	z	P	N	M	Z	p	N	M	z	p
C	42	+0.46	−0.63	.526	20	+0.70	−0.79	.427	17	+.11	−.23	.821
E	42	+6.47	−5.50	.000	17	+1.88	−1.80	.079	11	+.73	−.95	.344

M = mean change scores

Because there were no pretest differences between comparison and experimental groups on the Role Functioning Scale and because the Role Functioning Scale is an ordinal scale, the Mann-Whitney U test was used to examine differences among the comparison and experimental groups at each of the three posttests. The findings are summarized in Table 16. Comparison of scores revealed statistically significant findings at posttest 1 (n = 84, p = .0002), but nonsignificant findings at posttest 2 (n = 37, p = .256), and posttest 3 (n = 28, p = .090).

Within-group tests, using the Wilcoxon Matched-Pairs Signed-Ranks Test, were also conducted. The findings are summarized in Table 17. Examination of scores for the comparison group showed statistically significant findings from pretest to posttest 1 (n = 42, p = .003), but showed nonsignificant findings from posttest 1 to posttest 2 (n = 20, p = .219), and posttest 2 to posttest 3 (n = 17, p = .231). However, comparison of scores for the experimental group revealed statistically significant findings for all posttests including pretest to posttest 1 (n = 42, p = .000), posttest 1 to posttest 2 (n = 17, p = .006), and posttest 2 to posttest 3 (n = 11, p = .007).

Although both the comparison and experimental groups showed statistically significant level of change at posttest 1, the experimental group demonstrated a greater level of change. However, because both the comparison and experimental groups showed statistically significant findings at posttest 1, the level of change in individual roles in the

TABLE 16. Role Functioning Scale: Comparison of Posttest Findings Between Comparison and Experimental Groups

Posttest 1 (4 weeks)			Posttest 2 (8 weeks)			Posttest 3 (12 weeks)		
N	z	P	N	Z	p	N	z	p
84	−3.71	.0002	37	−1.13	.256	28	−1.69	.090

TABLE 17. Role Functioning Scale: Comparison of Posttest Findings Within Comparison and Experimental Groups

	Post 1 (4 weeks)				Post 2 (8 weeks)				Post 3 (12 weeks)			
	N	M	z	p	N	M	z	p	N	M	z	P
C	42	+1.71	−2.9	.003	20	+0.5	−1.2	.219	17	+1.53	−1.2	.231
E	42	+5.00	−5.6	.000	17	+1.3	−2.7	.006	11	+2.27	−2.7	.007

M = Mean change scores

Role Functioning Scale were examined. These results are summarized in Figure 1. The experimental group demonstrated greater levels of change in each of the four roles.

Findings from these tests indicate that the participants in the Role Development program demonstrated greater functioning in social roles than participants involved in the multidepartmental activity program at four, eight, and 12 weeks of treatment although the improvements at eight and 12 weeks were not statistically significant between groups. Additionally, participants in the comparison group demonstrated statistically significant improvement in social roles at four weeks although to a much lesser extent than the participants in the experimental group. A closer examination of each of the roles in the Role Functioning Scale at four weeks of treatment demonstrated that the participants in the experimental group showed a greater degree of change in all four roles.

REPEATED MEASURES ANALYSIS OF VARIANCE

The fourth hypothesis specifically addressed the effect of time on a participant's development of task skills, interpersonal skills, and roles, and was written as follows: The longer an individual participates in

FIGURE 1. Role Functioning Scale: Degree of Change in Individual Roles

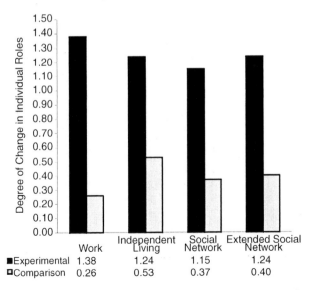

	Work	Independent Living	Social Network	Extended Social Network
■Experimental	1.38	1.24	1.15	1.24
□Comparison	0.26	0.53	0.37	0.40

treatment based on Role Development, the greater will the impact be on his development of social roles and the task and interpersonal skills associated with these roles. A repeated measures analysis of variance was used to analyze the effect of time.

Repeated measures analysis of variance is a statistical measure used to examine multiple observations of a scale over time and/or under different conditions (Green, Salkind, & Akey, 2000). In this study, repeated measures ANOVA was conducted to test for between-group differences (comparison and experimental groups) and within-group differences over time. Repeated measures ANOVA for between-group differences is entitled Multivariate Analysis and repeated measures ANOVA for within-group differences is entitled Tests of Within-Subjects Effects. The measurement of time consists of time elapsed over the 12 weeks of each aspect of the study with measurements at pretest, posttest 1 (4 weeks), posttest 2 (8 weeks) and posttest 3 (12 weeks). Repeated measures ANOVA was conducted independently with the Task Skills Scale, Interpersonal Skills Scale, and the Role Functioning Scale.

Box's Test of Equality of Covariance Matrices was conducted prior to the repeated measures ANOVA tests. "This statistic tests whether covariance matrices for the dependent variables are significantly different" (George & Mallery, 2000, p. 216). With this test it is preferable that the covariance matrices are not significantly different (p > .05). However, "this test is very sensitive, so just because it detects differences between the variance-covariance matrices does not necessarily mean that the F values are invalid" (George & Mallery, 2000, p. 217).

Multivariate analysis of variance was conducted to measure between-group effects over time. Because this is conducted only with the participants who completed all 12 weeks of the study, the number of participants is less than the number at pretest and posttest 1 and unequal for the comparison and experimental group. The number of participants for this measure is 17 for the comparison group and 11 for the experimental group.

In the tests of within-subjects effects, the within-subjects factor is time with four levels (pretest, 4, 8, and 12 weeks) and the dependent variable is the scores on each instrument at the four levels. In a within-subjects test, the sphericity assumption can be a problem. This assumption states that "correlations between all pairs of measurements are roughly the same. This means that measurements over several different times are not particularly robust to this assumption" (Sherry, 1997, p. 1). This problem is common in repeated measures over time. However, "the Greenouse-Gussier correction will fix the sphericity problem" (Sherry, 1997, p. 1). The Greenouse-Gussier correction was conducted in each of the tests of within-subjects effects.

Repeated Measures ANOVA–Role Functioning Scale

Box's Test of Equality of Covariance Matrices was conducted prior to the repeated measures ANOVA tests. This test was found to be not statistically significant at p = .06 (p > .05).

A multivariate repeated measures ANOVA was conducted with the factor being the two groups (comparison [n = 17] and experimental [n = 11]) over time (RFS pretest, posttest 1, posttest 2, and posttest 3) and the dependent variable being the Role Functioning Scale scores. The results for this test are presented in Table 18. The results for the ANOVA indicated a statistically significant between-group effect, Wilks's Λ = .689, F (3, 24) = 3.60, p = .028, eta squared = .31.

A test of within-subjects effect was conducted with the factor being time (RFS pretest, posttest 1, posttest 2, and posttest 3) and the dependent variable being the Role Functioning Scale scores. The results for this test are presented in Table 19. The results for the ANOVA indicated a statistically significant within-group effect for Time (main effect) (df = 3, F = 28.30, p = .000, eta squared = .52) and Time*Type (interaction effect) (df = 3, F = 4.742, p = .004, eta squared = .15). Interaction effect and mean scores for the Role Functioning Scale are presented in Figure 2.

TABLE 18. Role Functioning Scale: Multivariate Repeated Measures ANOVA for Four Time Periods

Effect Time*Type	Value	F	Hyp df	Error df	Sig.	Eta Squared
Wilks's Lambda	.689	3.60	3.00	24.00	.028	.31

TABLE 19. Role Functioning Scale: Within-Subjects Effect Repeated Measures ANOVA for Four Time Periods

Source	Df	F	Sig.	Eta Squared
Time Sphericity Assumed	3	28.30	.000	.521
Time*Type Sphericity Assumed	3	4.742	.004	.154
Error (Time) Sphericity Assumed	78	-	-	-

FIGURE 2. Interaction Effect and Mean Score: Role Functioning Scale

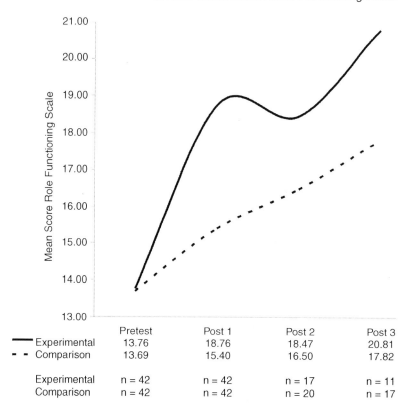

	Pretest	Post 1	Post 2	Post 3
—— Experimental	13.76	18.76	18.47	20.81
- - Comparison	13.69	15.40	16.50	17.82
Experimental	n = 42	n = 42	n = 17	n = 11
Comparison	n = 42	n = 42	n = 20	n = 17

Repeated Measures ANOVA–Task Skills Scale

Box's Test of Equality of Covariance Matrices was conducted prior to the repeated measures ANOVA tests. This was found to be statistically significant at p = .008 (p < .05). However, as mentioned above, "this test is very sensitive . . . differences between the variance-covariance matrices does not necessarily mean that the F values are invalid" (George & Mallery, 2000, p. 217).

A multivariate repeated measures ANOVA was conducted with the factor being the two groups (comparison [n = 17] and experimental [n = 11]) over time (TSS pretest, posttest 1, posttest 2, and posttest 3) and the dependent variable being the Task Skills Scale scores. The results for this test are presented in Table 20. The results for the ANOVA indicated a statistically significant between-group effect, Wilks's Λ = .682, F (3, 24) = 3.73, p = .025, eta squared = .31.

A test of within-subjects effect was conducted with the factor being time (TSS pretest, posttest 1, posttest 2, and posttest 3) and the dependent variable being the Task Skills Scale scores. The results for this test are presented in Table 21. The results for the ANOVA indicated a statistically significant within-group effect for Time (main effect) (df = 3, F = 8.807, p = .000, eta squared = .25) and Time*Type (interaction effect) (df = 3, F = 7.814, p = .000, eta squared = .23). Interaction effect and mean scores for the Task Skills Scale are presented in Figure 3.

Repeated Measures ANOVA–Interpersonal Skills Scale

Box's Test of Equality of Covariance Matrices was conducted prior to the repeated measures ANOVA tests. This was found to be not statistically significant at p = .448 (p > .05).

A multivariate repeated measures ANOVA was conducted with the factor being the two groups (comparison [n = 17] and experimental [n = 11]) over time (ISS pretest, posttest 1, posttest 2, and posttest 3) and the dependent variable being the Interpersonal Skills Scale scores. The results for this test are presented in Table 22. The results for the ANOVA indicated a statistically significant between-group effect, Wilks's Λ = .669, F (3, 24) = 3.96, p = .020, eta squared = .33.

TABLE 20. Task Skills Scale: Multivariate Repeated Measures ANOVA for Four Time Periods

Effect Time*Type	Value	F	Hypothesis df	Error df	Sig.	Eta Squared
Wilks's Lambda	.682	3.73	3.00	24.00	.025	.31

TABLE 21. Task Skills Scale: Within-Subjects Effect Repeated Measures ANOVA for Four Time Periods

Source	Df	F	Sig.	Eta Squared
Time Sphericity Assumed	3	8.807	.000	.253
Time*Type Sphericity Assumed	3	7.814	.000	.231
Error (Time) Sphericity Assumed	78	-	-	-

FIGURE 3. Interaction Effect and Mean Score: Task Skills Scale

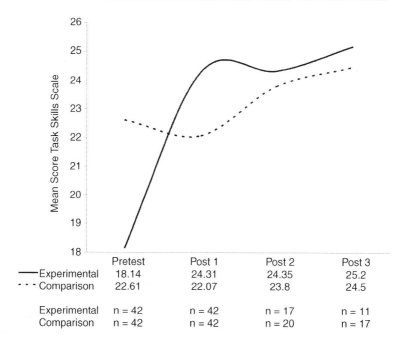

	Pretest	Post 1	Post 2	Post 3
——Experimental	18.14	24.31	24.35	25.2
- - - Comparison	22.61	22.07	23.8	24.5
Experimental	n = 42	n = 42	n = 17	n = 11
Comparison	n = 42	n = 42	n = 20	n = 17

TABLE 22. Interpersonal Skills Scale: Multivariate Repeated Measures ANOVA for Four Time Periods

Effect Time*Type	Value	F	Hypothesis df	Error df	Sig.	Eta Squared
Wilks's Lambda	.669	3.96	3.00	24.00	.020	.331

A test of within-subjects effect was conducted with the factor being time (TSS pretest, posttest 1, posttest 2, and posttest 3) and the dependent variable being the Interpersonal Skills Scale scores. The results for this test are presented in Table 23. The results of the ANOVA indicated a statistically significant within-group effect for Time (main effect) (df = 3, $F = 9.722$, p = .000, eta squared = .27) and Time*Type (interaction effect) (df = 3, $F = 6.779$, p = .000, eta squared = .20). Interaction effect and mean scores for the Interpersonal Skills Scale are presented in Figure 4.

TABLE 23. Interpersonal Skills Scale: Within-Subjects Effect Repeated Measures ANOVA for Four Time Periods

Source	df	F	Sig.	Eta Squared
Time Sphericity Assumed	3	9.722	.000	.272
Time*Type Sphericity Assumed	3	6.779	.000	.207
Error (Time) Sphericity Assumed	78	-	-	-

FIGURE 4. Interaction Effect and Mean Score: Interpersonal Skills Scale

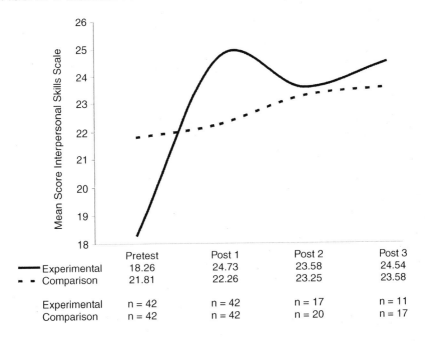

	Pretest	Post 1	Post 2	Post 3
—— Experimental	18.26	24.73	23.58	24.54
- - Comparison	21.81	22.26	23.25	23.58
Experimental	n = 42	n = 42	n = 17	n = 11
Comparison	n = 42	n = 42	n = 20	n = 17

Findings from these tests indicate that the participants in the Role Development program demonstrated greater functioning in task skills, interpersonal skills, and role functioning than participants involved in the multidepartmental activity program over the 12-week length of each group. Because repeated measures ANOVA only incorporates patients who participated for the entire length of each group (i.e., comparison group N = 17; experimental group, N = 11), the N is unequal and smaller in number. Nevertheless, statistically significant findings ranging from .028 to .000 were found with each test for both between-group and within-subject effects.

RELATIONSHIP BETWEEN TASK SKILLS SCALE, INTERPERSONAL SKILLS SCALE, AND THE ROLE FUNCTIONING SCALE

Although none of the hypotheses specifically addressed the relationship between task skills, interpersonal skills, and role functioning, the Principal Investigator believed this would be meaningful to assess given the assumption in Role Development that task skills and interpersonal skills are nested within social roles. A measurement of the relationship of these variables to one another would also be an important precursor to the MANCOVA.

To enact a role effectively, individuals need a repertoire of task and interpersonal skills (Black, 1976; Liberman et al., 1993; Mosey, 1986; Versluys, 1980). For example, an individual in the role of student would need task skills and interpersonal skills to participate in activities typical of a student (e.g., complete homework, interact with other students). Because Role Development views skills as the foundation of roles, correlations were conducted to determine if a relationship existed between the Task Skills Scale, the Interpersonal Skills Scale and the Role Functioning Scale. Correlations were conducted between pretest scores and posttest 1 scores on each of the three scales. Because all of these scales measure ordinal data, Spearman Correlation Coefficients are reported. The results are described in Table 24. Correlations between pretest scores for the comparison group ranged from .76-.86, and correlations for the posttest 1 scores for the comparison group ranged from .83-.89. Correlations between pretest scores for the experimental group ranged from .74-.80, and correlations for the posttest 1 scores for the experimental group ranged from .67-.88. Each one of the variables has some relationship with the other variable. This is not surprising considering that a premise in the theoretical base of Role Development is that task skills and interpersonal skills are nested within social roles (Schindler, 2002).

Multivariate Analysis of Covariance

Although none of the hypotheses specifically addressed assessing the effect of the Role Development program on a combined dependent vari-

TABLE 24. Correlation Coefficients Between Task Skills Scale, Interpersonal Skills Scale and the Role Functioning Scale for Comparison and Experimental Groups for Pretest and Posttest

Comparison Group								
	ISS Pre	ISS Pre	RFS Pre	RFS Pre	ISS Post 1	ISS Post 1	RFS Post 1	RFS Post 1
	C	p	C	P	C	p	C	P
TSS PRE	.867	.000	.760	.000				
ISS PRE			.765	.000				
TSS Post 1					.895	.000	.869	.000
ISS Post 1							.838	.000
Experimental Group								
	ISS Pre	ISS Pre	RFS Pre	RFS Pre	ISS Post 1	ISS Post 1	RFS Post 1	RFS Post 1
	C	p	C	P	C	p	C	P
TSS PRE	.804	.000	.745	.000				
ISS PRE			.785	.000				
TSS Post 1					.881	.000	.721	.000
ISS Post 1							.671	.000

C = correlation coefficient   p = level of significance

able (Task Skills Scale, Interpersonal Skills Scale, and the Role Functioning Scale) the Principal Investigator believed this would be meaningful to assess given the relationship among these variables. Therefore a multivariate analysis of covariance (MANCOVA) was conducted.

Multivariate analysis of covariance (MANCOVA) is a test to determine if "there are statistically significant mean differences among groups after adjusting the newly created dependent variable (a linear combination of all original dependent variables) for differences on one or more covariates" (Mertler & Vannatta, 2002, p. 137). MANCOVA tests that are conducted on samples of 20 or greater with only a few dependent variables will be sufficient to ensure robustness to violations of multivariate normality. Wilks's Lambda is commonly used as the MANCOVA statistic and was used for this test. MANCOVA is preferred to MANOVA when there are covariates. By incorporating the covariates into the analysis, the effects of these covariates can be removed, leaving a clearer picture of the effect of the independent variable on the dependent variables (Mertler & Vannatta, 2002).

A MANCOVA was conducted to determine if there are statistically significant mean differences in the combined dependent variable (Task Skills Scale, Interpersonal Skills Scale, Role Functioning Scale) between the comparison and experimental groups after removing the effects of pretest differences on the Task Skills Scale and Interpersonal Skills. Because there were pretest differences on the TSS and the ISS, the pretest scores on these scales were used as the covariates. The MANCOVA was conducted on the sample of 84 participants.

Box's Test of Equality of Covariance Matrices was conducted prior to the MANCOVA tests. This was found to be not statistically significant at p = .690 (p > .05).

The results for the MANCOVA revealed statistically significant differences between the comparison and experimental groups on the combined dependent variables, Wilks's $\Lambda = .687$, $F(3,77) = 11.70$, p < .001) (see Table 25).

Comparison Group–Clients Receiving Individual Attention

Every other client in the comparison group (50%) received up to 15 minutes of individual attention per week from each of the staff who had these participants in their groups. Staff were given a form indicating the name of the client to whom they should give the individual attention and directions on how to provide the individual attention. Clients who were lost through attrition were replaced. The purpose of 15 minutes of individual attention per week was to give equivalent amounts of individual

TABLE 25. Between-Subjects Effect MANCOVA for Comparison and Experimental Groups

Source	Dependent Variable	df	Mean Square	F	Sig.
ISS Pretest	RFS Post 1	1	37.652	3.631	.060
	ISS Post 1	1	103.375	6.375	.014
	TSS Post 1	1	35.055	1.795	.184
TSS Pretest	RFS Post 1	1	15.347	1.480	.227
	ISS Post 1	1	49.301	3.040	.085
	TSS Post 1	1	135.098	6.919	.010
Type of Group	RFS Post 1	1	372.908	35.963	.000
	ISS Post 1	1	259.424	15.998	.000
	TSS Post 1	1	337.554	17.287	.000

attention to these participants and to the participants in the experimental group. Participants in the experimental group also received 15 minutes of individual attention per week, but their 15 minutes of attention was focused on their progress within the Role Development intervention. This aspect of the research design raised two questions: (1) How do the participants receiving individual attention in the comparison group compare to those not receiving individual attention in the comparison group? and (2) Does individual attention or the experimental intervention cause a change in the dependent variables?

Upon completion of the study, the scores of the 21 clients receiving individual attention in the comparison group were analyzed. Thirteen of these participants (61%) demonstrated an increase in their scores on the Role Functioning Scale, seven participants (33%) demonstrated a decrease in scores, and one participant (4%) demonstrated no change in scores. This is in comparison to 25 of the 42 comparison group participants (60%) who showed an increase in their scores on the Role Functioning Scale. This demonstrates relatively no difference in posttest 1 scores between the comparison group participants receiving individual attention and those who did not receive individual attention. In contrast, 13 of these 21 participants (62%) receiving individual attention demonstrated a decrease in their scores on the Task Skills Scale and Interpersonal Skills Scale. This is in comparison to 23 of the 42 comparison group participants (55%) who showed a decrease in scores on the Task Skills Scale from pretest to posttest 1 and 19 of the 42 participants (45%) who showed a decrease in scores on the Interpersonal Skills Scale from pretest to posttest 1. Comparison group participants receiving individual attention actually received lower scores on the Task Skills Scale and the Interpersonal Skills Scale than those who did not receive individual attention. Therefore, results indicate that it was the experimental intervention that caused the change in task skills, interpersonal skills and role functioning.

Ten of these comparison group participants were discharged from the facility after posttest 1, leaving only 11 participants for the remaining two months of the study. Therefore, the data regarding differences among participants receiving individual attention (and those who did not receive individual attention) were analyzed only at posttest 1.

It should be noted, however, that when staff were asked to give individual attention in the format described above to the participants in the comparison group, the majority of staff stated that this would be no different than the way they typically interact with their patients in a given week. Therefore, all of the clients in the comparison group may have been receiving 15 minutes of individual attention per week.

ROLE CHECKLIST

An aspect of the third hypothesis addressed the Role Checklist and was written as follows: Adults diagnosed with schizophrenic disorders develop more social roles (as evidenced by a statistically significant improvement in scores on the Role Functioning Scale and a greater number of roles on the Role Checklist) when involved in individualized intervention based on Role Development in comparison to participation in a multidepartmental activity program.

The Role Checklist (Barris, Oakley, & Kielhofner, 1988; Oakley, 1981) is a self-report checklist that assesses an individual's ability to identify the roles in his or her life and the degree of satisfaction attributed to each role. Although results from the Role Checklist did contribute interesting and useful findings to the study, this instrument was not implemented as intended. The hypothesis addressing the Role Checklist stated that the participants involved in the Role Development program would develop more social roles as evidenced by a greater number of roles on the Role Checklist. Each participant in the study completed the Role Checklist during the pretest interview. However, at each of the posttest interviews, the participants did not select additional roles, but only commented on their progress, satisfaction, and continuation with the roles they selected at the pretest. Also, because the Role Checklist is a self-report checklist, each participant could choose between zero to four roles to develop during his participation in the study. This, coupled with attrition at each of the posttests, created a very unequal number of roles to be analyzed at each posttest. Hence, the quantitative findings do not directly address the hypothesis. Therefore, the findings from the Role Checklist that are most relevant to the hypothesis are described below.

The results of the Role Checklist begin with descriptive summary statistics for the comparison and experimental groups. Figure 5 provides a description of the total number of participants who selected each role. A few statistics of interest emerged from this description. For the worker role, although 75 participants identified this role as a past role, and 71 participants identified this role as a future role, only 39 participants stated that they wanted to develop this role during their current hospitalization. Although 69 participants identified friend as a past role, and 68 selected this as a future role, only 45 participants stated that they wanted to develop this role during their current hospitalization. Because the Role Checklist was completed during the pretest, some participants may have been too preoccupied with their psychiatric and legal problems to consider developing work, school, or friend roles at this early stage in their hospitalization.

The role of group member presented data different from the previous-mentioned roles. Forty-eight participants identified group member as a past and future role, but this number increased to 53 in the participants who identified group member as a role they want to develop during their current hospitalization.

Perhaps previous group treatment was limited for some of these participants, but they expected groups to be an aspect of their current treatment and identified it as a means to facilitate their treatment.

Despite the overall picture of a group of participants with severe and persistent mental illness, long psychiatric history, criminal charges, and low levels of education, more than half of the participants identified the

FIGURE 5. Role Checklist: Participant Choices During Program Study

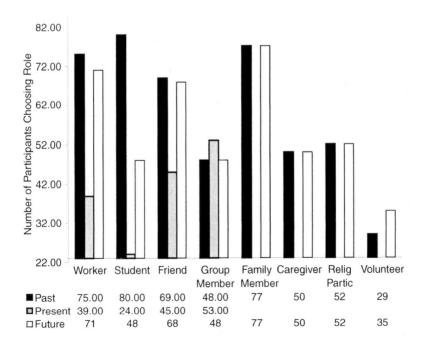

	Worker	Student	Friend	Group Member	Family Member	Caregiver	Relig Partic	Volunteer
■ Past	75.00	80.00	69.00	48.00	77	50	52	29
▨ Present	39.00	24.00	45.00	53.00				
□ Future	71	48	68	48	77	50	52	35

roles of caregiver, family member, and religious participant as roles they had in the past and would like to have in the future. A smaller number of participants identified volunteer as a role they had in the past (34%) and would like to have in the future (42%). It is understandable that this group of participants may not have had the skill or ability to volunteer nor the realistic opportunity in the future to do so given the demographic nature of this sample.

To determine if a relationship existed between the identification of a role as a past or future role and the selection of this role as a role to develop during the current hospitalization, correlations were conducted. Because the data regarding the identification or selection of a role are nominal data, nonparametric correlations were conducted. Correlations were conducted separately for the comparison group and the experimental group.

Results of the correlations are outlined in Tables 26 and 27. It is important to note that the selection of a role as a past and/or future role, or as a role to currently develop, occurred at the pretest for both groups. At this time, the groups differed only in the information they were given during the informed consent process. Neither group would have had participation in the intervention at this beginning stage of the process.

For the comparison group, the only statistically significant correlations existed between: (1) the selection of friend as a future role and friend as a current role; and (2) the selection of a group member as a past and future role with the selection of group member as a current role. Be-

TABLE 26. Comparison Group: Correlations Between Roles in the Past/Future with Role in the Present

	Student–Present		Worker–Present		Friend–Present		Group Member–Present	
Role	C	p	C	p	C	p	C	p
Student–Past	.144	.360						
Student–Future	.217	.166						
Worker–Past			.288	.064				
Worker–Future			−.021	.890				
Friend–Past					.265	.090		
Friend–Future					.395	.010		
Grp Mem–Past							.619	.000
Grp Mem–Future							.611	.000

C = correlation; p = p value

TABLE 27. Experimental Group: Correlations Between Roles in the Past/Future with Role in the Present

Role	Student–Present C	Student–Present p	Worker–Present C	Worker–Present p	Friend–Present C	Friend–Present p	Group Member–Present C	Group Member–Present p
Student–Past	#	#						
Student–Future	.673	.000						
Worker–Past			−.046	.733				
Worker–Future			.333	.033				
Friend–Past					.301	.058		
Friend–Future					.455	.003		
Grp Mem–Past							.368	.016
Grp Mem–Future							.068	.667

C = correlation; p = p value; # = coefficient cannot be computed

cause treatment is provided in a group format in the rehabilitation wing, participants in the comparison group may have expected to work on a group member role.

For the experimental group, statistically significant correlations existed in the student, worker, friend, and group member roles. However, only in the friend role were correlations statistically significant for both the past and future friend role with the current friend role. Perhaps through the explanation of their involvement in Role Development during the informed consent process, participants realized they would be encouraged and assisted with these roles, and therefore identified them as roles they would like to develop during their current hospitalization.

The fact that there were more statistically significant correlations between selection of past, present, and future roles for participants in the Role Development program as compared to participants in the multidepartmental activity program, does support the hypothesis that participants involved in the Role Development program would select a greater number of roles on the Role Checklist (see Tables 26 and 27).

CONCLUSION

This chapter began with demographic data on the sample followed by results of the pretests. Then, each of the four research hypotheses was addressed through the findings of the tests of the significance of the intervention. After the major findings, quantitative data were presented on the staff participating in the training and implementation of Role Development, followed by qualitative data on staff and patient perceptions of the effectiveness of the intervention.

The examination of demographic data revealed that there were no differences in characteristics between participants in the experimental and control groups. Examination of pretest differences between the two groups revealed that although there were no statistically significant pretest differences on the Role Functioning Scale, statistically significant pretest differences did exist on the Task Skills Scale and Interpersonal Skills Scale.

To address the four research hypotheses, statistical tests were conducted first on each scale individually (Task Skills Scale, Interpersonal Skills Scale, and Role Functioning Scale) followed by statistical tests that addressed confounding variables, repeated measures of analysis, and multivariates. Then, the Role Checklist was examined followed by quantitative and qualitative data on the staff participating in the Role Development program.

Overall, data analysis on the three scales indicated that participants in the experimental group showed greater improvement in the development of task skills, interpersonal skills, and role functioning in comparison to participants in the comparison group. This held true for a subgroup of the comparison group (one-half of the participants in the comparison group) who received weekly individual attention in addition to the multidepartmental activity program. This aspect of the design was to control for the effect of individual attention and to determine if it was the intervention, rather than individual attention alone, that caused the positive change. The Role Checklist, a self-report checklist, offered some data regarding the participants' perception of their roles, but meaningful data from this instrument were limited due to circumstances of the program's location.

Chapter 7

Evaluating the Effectiveness of Role Development: Qualitative Data

QUALITATIVE FINDINGS

This study included two areas of qualitative findings. Current research trends describe that it is efficacious to include both quantitative and qualitative findings in a study. Qualitative findings promote further understanding of quantitative findings (Bailey, 1998; Depoy & Gitlin, 1998). In this study, qualitative findings were used for this purpose and to further understand the perceptions of the staff and patients involved in this study. Focus groups were conducted with the rehabilitation staff implementing Role Development and these are described in Chapter 9. Additionally, patient participants who completed 12 weeks in the comparison or experimental group were interviewed at the conclusion of their participation in the study. These qualitative findings are discussed in this chapter. To conduct the qualitative analysis, the Principal Investigator identified patterns and systematically organized these into trends, topics, and categories, and noted exceptions to these patterns (Bailey, 1998; Depoy & Gitlin, 1998). Although the hypotheses did not specifically address the collection of qualitative data, this information was collected to enhance and add to the quantitative findings.

[Haworth co-indexing entry note]: "Evaluating the Effectiveness of Role Development: Qualitative Data." Schindler, Victoria P. Co-published simultaneously in *Occupational Therapy in Mental Health* (The Haworth Press, Inc.) Vol. 20, No. 3/4, 2004, pp. 105-109; and: *Occupational Therapy in Forensic Psychiatry: Role Development and Schizophrenia* (Victoria P. Schindler) The Haworth Press, Inc., 2004, pp. 105-109. Single or multiple copies of this article are available for a fee from The Haworth Document Delivery Service [1-800-HAWORTH, 9:00 a.m. - 5:00 p.m. (EST). E-mail address: docdelivery@haworthpress.com].

http://www.haworthpress.com/web/OTMH
© 2004 by The Haworth Press, Inc. All rights reserved.
Digital Object Identifier: 10.1300/J004v20n03_07

PATIENT INTERVIEWS

The Principal Investigator interviewed patient participants who completed 12 weeks in the comparison or experimental group and were still in the facility at the conclusion of their respective aspect of the study. Seventeen patients completed 12 weeks in the comparison group, but only 12 of these patients were still in the facility at the conclusion of data collection for the comparison group. Although 11 patients completed 12 weeks in the experimental group, only 10 of these patients were still in the facility at the conclusion of data collection for the experimental group. Therefore, there were 12 patients who participated in interviews regarding the comparison group (N = 12) and 10 patients who participated in interviews regarding the experimental group (N = 10). All patients were asked the following questions:

1. Tell me about the groups you have been in. What about them have you liked or disliked?
2. What about the groups have been helpful?
3. How have the groups helped you to prepare for when you leave here?
4. What do you recommend to do differently?

Comparison Group

In response to the first question, two categories of response occurred. Eight patients (66%) indicated that the activities in the groups were something they liked. Seven patients (58%) stated that they like the rehabilitation staff. One of these patients commented, "most of the staff are helpful and therapeutic."

In response to the second question, regarding the helpfulness of the groups, two categories of response emerged. All 12 patients (100%) indicated that the groups served as a means to distract them from their problems or occupy their time while in the hospital. One of the patients stated that it made this time of his life "more bearable" while another stated that the programs help him to "kill time." Another patient stated, "It takes my mind off of things so I don't have time to think about the negative things." Two patients stated that the groups give them an opportunity to gain respect for others and their problems and an opportunity to help others.

The third question addressed the patient's ability to ascertain if he learned anything in the groups that would help him once he leaves the facility. Two categories of response emerged, both of them indicating that the patient did not feel as though he learned anything that could help him once he leaves the facility. Eight patients (66%) could not give any examples of something they learned that could be generalized to their next living environment. Three patients (25%) specifically answered "nothing." One of these patients added, "Nothing in these groups ties into anything outside of here." Another patient added, "It only occupies my time; it doesn't address my problems."

The fourth question asked the patient for recommendations. Three patients (25%) had no suggestions, but all of the other patients (75%) had at least one suggestion. Some of these suggestions included "better work opportunities, programs to help you identify your problems, more discussion groups, programs to help you adjust to being here."

Three major themes emerged from the interviews with the patients in the comparison group: (1) the rehabilitation programs are helpful to the extent that they provide a distraction and a means to occupy time, but they do not provide a means to learn necessary skills; (2) the patients did not experience the development of any skills that they could use to improve their lives in their future environments; and (3) the patients had some concrete ideas and suggestions to improve the existing program to better meet their needs.

Experimental Group

In response to the first question, four categories of response occurred. As with the comparison group, two groups of patients indicated that the activities (60%) and rehabilitation staff (30%) were things that they liked about the program. However, in contrast to the comparison group, three patients (30%) stated that they liked learning skills and four patients (40%) indicated that they liked learning roles. One of these patients stated, "It has helped me prepare for work and to find friends."

In response to indicating what was helpful about the groups, three categories of response emerged. Four patients (40%) indicated that they had learned new skills, specifically in dealing with frustration. Three patients each (30%) indicated that it was helpful to be able to talk with staff one-on-one, and that they were able to increase their comfort in socializing with others.

In response to the third question, which addressed the patient's ability to ascertain if he learned anything in the groups that would help him once he leaves the facility, three categories of response emerged. Three patients (30%) described roles they have gained that will transfer to their next environment. One of these patients stated, "It will help me transition from being a student here to a student in the community." Another patient stated, "It has helped me to be more outspoken and to find friends." Six patients (50%) indicated that they increased their skills, and their description of skills formed three subcategories. All six patients stated that they improved their "work" skills, such as their ability to focus on and successfully complete their work. These two skills are examples of task skills. Three patients (30%) indicated that they have increased their coping skills, specifically their ability to positively deal with frustration. One of these patients stated, "By being able to come up with ways to deal with frustrations, it has helped me personally and will help me to be successful when I leave." Two patients (20%) cited interpersonal skills they have learned. One of these patients stated, "It prepares me to better deal with and respond to people."

In response to the last question regarding suggestions and recommendations, three patients (30%) stated that they are happy with the current program and could not add any other suggestions. Another patient suggested that this type of program be used in the prison settings. One patient asked if his friend could be in the study because "You get more help and attention if you are a patient in the study."

Two major themes emerged from the interviews of the patients in the experimental group: (1) patients were able to identify skills (specifically task and interpersonal skills) and roles they learned that uniquely addressed their needs and situations; (2) patients were able to identify a link between the learning of these skills and their ability to transfer this learning to future life situations.

Analysis of Findings Between Comparison and Experimental Groups

Both groups indicated that the rehabilitation program was a positive aspect of their hospitalization. However, for the comparison group this was primarily a productive use of time, while the patients in the experimental group could cite specific skills and roles they learned through their participation in the program. Also, the patients in the comparison group could not identify any long-term benefits of their participation in the multidepartmental activity program, while the patients in the experimental group were able to describe specific ways in which skills and roles could transfer to other life situations. Finally, the patients in the comparison group were able to offer concrete, meaningful suggestions to improve their program, and some of these suggestions focused on addressing roles and skills. It is hoped that a program based on Role Development would be able to address these suggestions.

CONCLUSION

Patients involved in the study reported contrasts between the interventions in the comparison and experimental groups. The participants in the Role Development program described the way in which they were able to develop roles and skills and remarked about the overall improvement in important aspects of their lives.

Chapter 8

Case Studies

Four case studies representing the application of Role Development will be presented in this chapter.

PAUL

A case study involving a client, Paul, was introduced in Chapter 1. For the purpose of convenience for the reader, the introductory information is repeated here followed by information on assessment and intervention.

Paul was a single, 20-year-old male, of Italian and African American descent. He was incarcerated following an altercation with his father and at the jail appeared to be responding to internal stimuli. Paul had resided with his parents and younger brother and sister ages 19 and 15 respectively. Both parents worked at a factory.

Paul completed the 11th grade at a Technical Institute and was a few months into 12th grade when he started to become withdrawn, isolative and paranoid. He refused to attend school and became more reclusive at home. In a short time he quit school and did not earn a high school diploma or a GED. He had one job as a busboy at a chain restaurant, but he quickly became suspicious of others and was absent from work. After only a few weeks he was fired for absenteeism. He began to argue with his parents more as their frustration with him grew.

[Haworth co-indexing entry note]: "Case Studies." Schindler, Victoria P. Co-published simultaneously in *Occupational Therapy in Mental Health* (The Haworth Press, Inc.) Vol. 20, No. 3/4, 2004, pp. 111-122; and: *Occupational Therapy in Forensic Psychiatry: Role Development and Schizophrenia* (Victoria P. Schindler) The Haworth Press, Inc., 2004, pp. 111-122. Single or multiple copies of this article are available for a fee from The Haworth Document Delivery Service [1-800-HAWORTH, 9:00 a.m. - 5:00 p.m. (EST). E-mail address: docdelivery@haworthpress.com].

Paul's family denied any history of alcohol or substance abuse or mental illness or legal problems. Paul denied any history of physical or sexual abuse. Paul also denied any history of substance abuse. He stated that he had tried alcohol but denied using it on a regular basis. He denied blackouts and denied using marijuana, cocaine, heroin, or other drugs. Records suggest that he might have used marijuana in the past but he denied such use. He had never been referred to, or treated in, a drug rehabilitation facility.

Paul had difficulty believing that he may have symptoms of schizophrenia. He repeatedly stated his belief that he does not need to take medications. He reported that the medication has no impact on him stating, "I feel the same with medication as without medication." In addition to the growing problems Paul was experiencing at home, Paul also stated he didn't have any friends or anyone with whom he could confide or talk.

Paul reported that his current legal problems resulted from an "argument" with his father. He stated that he was lying on the couch with his eyes closed, and his father was talking to him about getting a job and not lying around the house. Reportedly, his father threw a book at him, and "I started yelling at him." His mother and brother apparently tried to break up the fight. The police were called, arrested Paul, and charged him with harassment. Records indicate that such altercations have occurred in the past.

Paul's family and the police subsequently dropped all charges. However, Paul's family did not want him to return home. They stated he could only return home when he was settled in a job.

Application of Role Development to Assessment and Intervention

Upon initial assessment, Paul was observed in groups and he participated in a structured interview. The four assessments were completed, and Paul was given the following ratings: Task Skills Scale: 22 (mean 2.7); Interpersonal Skills Scale: 22 (mean 2.7); and the Role Functioning Scale: 14 (marginal). During the interview, Paul described that in the month prior to admission he was "zoning and spacing out." He said that he began to think about a job but his life was confusing and boring. He couldn't name any friends. Paul also completed the Role Checklist. Although he listed several roles he had in the past (student, worker, caregiver, friend, family member, religious participant) and several of these that he would like to have in the future, he did not view any of these roles as active in the present. He claimed to be "somewhat satisfied" with the majority of these roles. Paul initially was reluctant to identify any roles to address at the hospital because he just planned to "go home and help around the house." However, Paul's parents were adamant that Paul could not return home if he did not have a plan to work or attend school. Paul was reluctant to hear this information, but when reminded that he would probably feel better if he had some type of structure and plan for his life upon discharge, he agreed to pursue roles of student, worker, friend, and group member. Because he was unsure if he should work or try to obtain a GED, he decided to pursue the roles of student and worker to determine which role he preferred.

For the first week Paul needed a lot of support and encouragement to participate in any of the groups. He was very quiet, isolative, and gave only brief responses to questions. Staff reported that he had difficulty engaging in tasks and his work was slow, but when he did complete tasks, his work was "excellent." Paul was complimented on his accomplishments. Staff and Paul collaboratively set goals for Paul to complete his willingness to engage in tasks, to increase his comfort with peers, and to cooperate as a member of a group. All of these goals would be addressed within the roles described above.

By the second week in the program it was becoming clear that Paul had many strengths in his task skills but limitations in interpersonal skills. He preferred to work alone and demonstrated few limitations in cognitive skills. He was slowly increasing his concentration to tasks and could follow multi-step directions. Often, he was able to problem solve independently. Staff commented to him that the "thinking" skills he was demonstrating in groups are the same type of skills he would need to be successful in the roles of student and worker in the community. Interpersonally, Paul was still struggling. He would participate in tasks with the therapist when invited to do so, but was hesitant to participate with his peers. His verbal interactions were still limited and only initiated interactions with the therapists.

By the third week in the program, his willingness to participate in tasks increased to a greater variety of tasks. He worked independently in assembly-line type of vocational tasks and creative writing. He was able to identify himself as a student and worker. Now it was time to increase the focus on the roles of friend and group member. Although his socialization with peers was still limited, he did initiate conversation with staff and his interactions were appropriate. Staff reminded Paul that this type of interaction he was having with staff could be transferred to his interactions with peers. Staff and Paul continued to pursue goals related to increasing his comfort with his peers and as a group member.

One staff member personally invited Paul to participate in activities in the gym. The staff member would approach Paul, walk a few laps around the gym with him, and then invited him to play volleyball with him and a small group of patients. Paul was hesitant but did agree. At first he would play for a few minutes, but this increased as time went on. Paul and the staff member spoke of how volleyball is an example of an ordinary type of activity that a person does with friends or as a member of a group. Paul was able to see that by participating in an activity with others, he was able to be comfortable as a member of a group.

Paul remained in the program for two additional weeks. During this time his productivity in the vocational tasks increased to above average work. Paul was able to work the full one-hour period on school related tasks and had conversations with staff as to whether he should pursue his GED or look for a job upon discharge. He would stop staff in the hall and talk with them. With help from staff, he was able to work collaboratively with another peer in his groups and continued to participate in the volleyball games. Overall, his affect was much brighter and his optimism for the future emerged.

Prior to discharge Paul was reevaluated on the same four assessments described above (Task Skills Scale, Interpersonal Skills Scale, the Role Functioning Scale, and the Role Checklist). Paul demonstrated an increase in functioning in all three scales completed by the independent rater and was given the following ratings: Task Skills Scale: 29 (mean 3.6); Interpersonal Skills Scale: 29 (mean 3.6); and the Role Functioning Scale: 16 (moderate). During the interview, Paul reported that he was working, using the computers and that he was doing "pretty good" during the last month. In the follow-up to the Role Checklist, he reported that he was either somewhat satisfied or very satisfied with the roles he developed during his hospital stay, and that he had a "very good level of performance" in each of these roles.

Paul was transferred to a state psychiatric hospital where he could continue his involvement in therapeutic programs with eventual return to his own home or placement in a group home. Paul's plan was to continue to work toward his GED so that he could pursue a greater variety of work options in the future.

HUBERT

Hubert was a 44-year-old man who was sent to the facility after completing 27 years in prison for murder. He went into prison at age 17. He did not complete high school, was never married, and had no children. He maintained contact with his father and planned to live with him upon discharge. While in prison he received over 100 disciplinary charges prior to being diagnosed with schizophrenia. Once diagnosed and compliant with psychotropic medications (5 years prior to release from prison), he received no further disciplinary charges. While in prison he worked for a few months in an auto body shop, but otherwise he claimed he "isolated myself" and "minded my own business." He was referred to this facility upon release from prison for further treatment of his psychiatric illness before return to the community.

When he arrived he was angry about being sent to the facility. He stated he was under the impression he was being released to the community until he was told otherwise at his discharge interview. He agreed to participate in the Role Development program and attend groups, but said he would just be an observer. He spoke about being in prison and what it had taught him. He said that initially he tried to beat it, but then learned to just keep to himself, and mind his own business. Now he was hesitant to become involved in anything. Although he was angry, he was also a little overwhelmed about his return to the community. When he went into prison he was a teenager, now he was an adult man. He had never worked nor maintained any type of household. So much had changed in society during the 27 years he was in prison. This overwhelmed him. He was somewhat comforted by the fact that now he could begin to work on roles that would be required once he returned to the community.

Application of Role Development to Assessment and Intervention

Upon initial assessment, Hubert was observed in groups and he participated in a structured interview. The four assessments were completed, and Hubert was given the following ratings: Task Skills Scale: 21 (mean 2.6); Interpersonal Skills Scale: 20 (mean 2.5); and the Role Functioning Scale: 9 (limited). During the interview, Hubert described the time he had spent in prison. He said he spent most of his time listening to the radio, watching TV. He described his life as "bad."

He listed several roles he had in the past–most of them prior to his years in prison (student, worker, friend, family member, religious participant, group member)–and all of the roles that he would like to have in the future (except student). He claimed to be "somewhat satisfied" or "very satisfied" with his past performance in these roles. Hubert initially was reluctant to identify any roles to address at the hospital, but realizing he had some anxiety about returning to the community, he selected friend and group member as roles with which to begin.

During his first week in the program, Hubert demonstrated difficulties in both task and interpersonal skills. He had difficulty engaging in tasks, maintaining concentration, and attending to details. With others, he had difficulty interacting with his peers and cooperating as a member of a group. Staff set goals with Hubert to concentrate on these areas. They planned to establish a trusting relationship with Hubert, explore his interests in order to offer a variety of activities, and offer activities that initially required minimal cooperation.

Hubert had a slow start in the program. He complained of medication side effects. He was referred to his physician and his medication was adjusted. He reported improvement. However, he remained quiet and isolative.

Staff approached Hubert individually. It was discovered that he liked ping-pong. He was invited to play a game with staff. It was observed that he talked readily when involved in this game. Another staff member invited him to play Scrabble in a small group. It was also observed that conversation flowed more freely for him when involved in this type of activity. Staff commented on this to Hubert. Staff encouraged Hubert to see that he might be more comfortable making friends or being part of a group if he can do so through activities he enjoys. Staff and Hubert began to brainstorm activities that he could incorporate into life upon his return to the community.

During the third week of his participation in the program, it was noted that he was "maintaining concentration, opening up, and interacting with a few peers." During his final week in the program, he wrote a poem in the occupational therapy group, recited the poem, and submitted it for publication in the hospital newsletter. This was the first accomplishment of this type that he received in his life. He and his therapist spoke about this demonstration of his role as a group member and the task and interpersonal skills that were involved in this success. The occupational therapist pointed out to Hubert that these are the same types of skills basic to success in all types of tasks and interactions.

Although staff continued to report that he was more sociable, there was still some hesitancy in his involvement with peers. However, overall his level of participation and interaction increased greatly in his four weeks in the program. Prior to discharge he reported to the staff that the groups made him feel like he is "somebody."

Prior to discharge Hubert was reevaluated on the same four assessments described above (Task Skills Scale, Interpersonal Skills Scale, the Role Functioning Scale, and the Role Checklist). Hubert demonstrated great improvement in all of the scales completed by the independent rater and was given the following ratings: Task Skills Scale: 29 (mean 3.5); Interpersonal Skills Scale: 29 (mean 3.6); and the Role Functioning Scale: 15 (marginal). During the interview, Hubert reported that he was "going to classes, playing cards, drawing, and going to rehab activities." He stated that he was "somewhat able to perform" his roles of friend and group member. Although he knew he had a long road ahead, he seemed as if the skills and roles he developed during his hospitalization boosted his confidence to return to life in the community.

GEORGE

George was a 35-year-old male admitted to the facility after completing a 12-year sentence for Robbery and Aggravated Assault in a state prison. He had a history of anxiety attacks and depression, but had received no previous psychiatric treatment. Prior to his release from prison he reported hearing voices. He was diagnosed with Psychotic Disorder NOS and was prescribed antipsychotic and antidepressive medication. Prior to his incarceration he worked in roofing, plumbing and construction. He was divorced and had a 9th grade education.

On admission to the facility he was angry that he was not released to the community. He didn't believe he needed to be in the hospital. Within the first week he was in two altercations. He had to be restrained and placed in the quiet room. He became threatening to the security staff.

Once George was calm and able to attend the rehabilitation unit, he agreed to participate in the study. However, he believed he didn't really need any assistance with roles and that he could assume his roles automatically upon return to the community. He stated he didn't want to be friends with anyone because "They all have a lot of problems."

Application of Role Development to Assessment and Intervention

Upon initial assessment, George was observed in groups and he participated in a structured interview. The four assessments were completed, and George was given the following ratings: Task Skills Scale: 24 (mean 3.0); Interpersonal Skills Scale: 32 (mean 4.0); and the Role Functioning Scale: 20 (moderate). During the initial interview, George stated that he recently spent 23 or 24 hours per day in his cell in the prison.

He listed all of the roles on the Role Checklist as roles he had in the past and would like to have in the future. He claimed to be "very satisfied" with all of the roles with the exception of volunteer ("somewhat satisfied"). He listed the worker role and the group member role as roles he would like to pursue during the hospital stay.

For the first week in the program, George was observed by the rehabilitation staff to be somewhat hyperactive and possibly paranoid around others. He rushed through tasks without appropriate attention to detail. He frequently changed tasks, left tasks uncompleted, and worked so fast that quality was sacrificed. He was resistive to feedback and constructive criticism. He seemed uncomfortable with his peers. He was unable to carry on a casual conversation with others and seemed suspicious. Staff and George collaboratively set goals in the areas of task and interpersonal skills. These goals included: maintain concentration, attend to details, work with an appropriate rate of performance, cooperate as a member of a group and improve interaction with peers. Although George wanted to work in preparation for a worker role in the future, staff believed that George's current difficulty would impede success in a worker role.

George participated in the program for eight weeks after the initial assessments were completed. During the first week of the program George was observed to continue to rush through activities and make mistakes. Staff spoke with him as soon as this would occur, and he seemed to be able to adjust his work speed for at least a brief period of time. George was also noted to separate himself from group members. Staff noted "he sets himself apart" or that he monopolized group conversations or blurted unkind remarks. Staff spoke with him about the effect of these behaviors and the impact they would have on a successful role as a group member. Staff equated it to getting along with friends, co-workers, etc., in the community. Together they spoke of groups with which George is involved now and would be involved in the future (e.g., family, work, outpatient groups), and the consequences that this type of behavior could have. Staff and George agreed that they would set up activities in which he could practice working cooperatively with one other group member.

During the next few weeks George was noted to make slow but consistent progress. Staff noted that he "demonstrated improvements in slowing down and focusing on one thing at a time, but he is still impulsive at times." He was observed to be more responsive to feedback and had higher quality work when given one-to-one attention and consistent feedback. Progress in the area of interpersonal skills and group behavior was a little slower. Although he still preferred to work individually, he did respond to a suggestion to assist a fellow patient who had a physical disability. He seemed comfortable in this role, but had limited interaction with other group members. Near the end of this second phase in the program, group members supportively confronted George about his behavior (can be aloof and demanding) under the supervision of staff. The occupational therapist reported that "All comments were appropriate and George seemed to have gotten the message."

It was at approximately this point in his treatment that George participated in the four week reevaluation. He was reevaluated on the same four assessments described above (Task Skills Scale, Interpersonal Skills Scale, the Role Functioning Scale, and the Role Checklist). Although staff and George reported progress from the time of the initial assessments, the ratings given by the independent rater represented minimal change: Task Skills Scale: 26 (mean 3.2); Interpersonal Skills Scale: 31 (mean 3.8); and the Role Functioning Scale: 20 (moderate). During the interview, George reported that he was "going to rehab" and "doing great." He reported that he had made some friends. He also reported that he was "somewhat satisfied" with his roles, but that he didn't reach his goals yet.

It seemed as though that point was a turning point for George. He began to seriously consider and incorporate the feedback given to him by the staff and his peers. He began to participate more and become more helpful in the groups. His interactions were calmer and more positive. He took on the role of friend with an elderly, disabled peer and transported this peer to his groups in his wheelchair. He requested a work program and it was granted. Staff and George both agreed that he had developed the necessary task and interpersonal skills to be successful in a work situation.

In work he was able to learn the job quickly and in three weeks was promoted to a foreman position. He still had episodes of blurting out hostilities toward others, but these were less often. When they occurred, staff (and patients) would work with him to help him identify the negative consequences of his behavior. He became more accepting of this feedback. George was readily able to identify the progress he made as a group member and worker. He was also able to see that although he initially had no desire to form friendships, he was able to become a friend to several peers and enjoyed this role.

Prior to discharge George was reevaluated on the same four assessments described above (Task Skills Scale, Interpersonal Skills Scale, the Role Functioning Scale, and the Role Checklist). George was given the following ratings: Task Skills Scale: 32 (mean 4.0); Interpersonal Skills Scale: 26 (mean 3.2); and the Role Functioning Scale: 20 (moderate). These scores reflect an improvement in Task Skills, an ability to maintain the score in Role Functioning, and a decrease in score (6 points from initial) on the Interpersonal Skills Scale. Despite this decrease in scores in the Interpersonal Skills Scale from the independent rater, staff reported that George demonstrated great improvements in task and interpersonal skills. They reported that although there were periods of time when he could still be impulsive in tasks and interactions (the independent rater may have observed George during one of these times), these episodes were much less in number and he was more able to recognize and correct his behavior. During the pre-discharge interview, George reported that he was "working in horticulture and the workshop" and that he met several friends that he planned to remain in contact with once he was discharged. He stated that he was promoted to foreman in the workshop and that he was "very satisfied" with his roles and that he had achieved "very good level of performance."

George was discharged to live with his sister and brother-in-law. His brother-in-law arranged for him to work in a meat packaging facility. He has since written to the patients whom he befriended and appeared to be doing well.

GREG

Greg was a 35-year-old male admitted to the facility after being found Not Guilty by Reason of Insanity for robbery. Greg had a long history of psychiatric illness and had been hospitalized at least five times in the eight years prior to this admission. Prior to the arrest that led to this admission, Greg had been homeless. He had worked in the past as a truck driver and in a factory, but was unemployed during the time he was homeless. He had attended high school but did not complete his high school courses or obtain a GED. He was never married but had three children with whom he currently had no contact.

When Greg arrived at the facility he alternated between being quiet and guarded and being aggressive. He was diagnosed with schizoaffective disorder and placed on antipsycotic medication. Although a little unsure of how the treatment could benefit him, he agreed to participate in the study.

Application of Role Development to Assessment and Intervention

As with all of the participants, Greg was observed in groups and he participated in a structured interview for the initial assessment. The four assessments were completed, and Greg was given the following ratings: Task Skills Scale: 22 (mean 2.7); Interpersonal Skills Scale: 19 (mean 2.3); and the Role Functioning Scale: 17 (moderate). During the initial interview, Greg reported that he spent the last three years at a county jail. He said he had some opportunities to socialize with others at the jail. On the Role Checklist, with the exception of volunteer and religious participant, Greg listed all of the roles as roles he had in the past and would like to have in the future. He claimed to be "very satisfied" with all of the roles with the exception of friend ("somewhat satisfied"). He listed four roles to address during his hospital stay: worker, student, group member, and friend.

Greg participated in the program for 12 weeks. For the first week in the program, Greg was observed by the rehabilitation staff to have areas of need in task and interpersonal skills and in the four roles in which he had interest. With tasks he was observed to have difficulty concentrating and organizing tasks in a logical manner. His rate of performance was slow. Interpersonally, he had difficulty initiating verbal interactions and communicating accurately and expressing himself clearly (he made some delusional statements). He was unable to initiate friendships within the friend role and was uncomfortable working with others in a group situation. Although he stated that he would like to work, staff felt as though he needed to make some improvements to be successful at work. When he and staff discussed his strengths and needs, goals were set to increase his concentration and organization of tasks, increase his comfort and appropriateness in his conversations, initiate a friendship, and increase his comfort in group situations.

During his first weeks in the program, staff reported that although Greg stated that he wanted to make friends with others, he still vacillated between being quiet and guarded and then angry at times. One staff member reported that he "fades in and out." In one-to-one conversations it was noted that he verbalized fantasy or delusional material particularly focused on ninjas. An art therapist used this interest in fantasy to encourage Greg to participate in tasks. He agreed to draw superheroes. The art therapist introduced him to a few types of mediums (e.g., pastels, paints) and Greg was able to increase his concentration and organization through this activity. He took pride in this work so he worked carefully. The therapist and Greg spoke of how this task has similarities to other tasks and that if he can concentrate and do well on this, he could apply the same skills to tasks within other roles.

At about this point Greg participated in the four-week reevaluation. He was noted to obtain the following scores which reflected improvement in all areas evaluated by the independent rater: Task Skills Scale: 26 (mean 3.2); Interpersonal Skills Scale: 26 (mean 3.2); and the Role Functioning Scale: 20 (moderate). During the interview, Greg noted that, "It has been better since I got here," and felt that he was satisfied with his progress. A decision was made that he would begin to concentrate more on school work as he was feeling that his ability to focus on tasks was improving.

During the next phase of his treatment he increased his interest and involvement in school work. He wanted to make preliminary steps toward pursing a GED. He was particularly interested in math. Although his attention and motivation were good, his math skills were basic. He required much individual assistance that the teacher was not always able to give. Also, he still preferred to work alone, and working on math problems independently would not help him to increase his comfort with others. Together the teacher and Greg discussed this dilemma and the impact this had on his desire to develop student, friend, and group member roles. In discussing this the teacher suggested that Greg work with another patient in the class. This patient had excellent math skills but also tended to be a loner. If they worked as a pair, they could each address their goals. Both patients agreed to this and worked together for one hour daily for the duration of Greg's time in the program. Both were continually provided with positive feedback on their development of respective roles. Instead of adding a worker role, Greg decided to increase his student role by adding a second course during the day (English).

Greg was reevaluated at eight and 12 weeks. His scores on the assessments maintained or increased at both intervals. At the final evaluation he was noted to have obtained the following scores: Task Skills Scale: 29 (mean 3.6); Interpersonal Skills Scale: 26 (mean 3.2); and the Role Functioning Scale: 21 (adequate). During the final interview, he noted that he was very satisfied with all of his roles and rated himself as having a "very good level of performance."

Chapter 9

Response of the Rehabilitation Staff to Role Development

THE PARTICIPATING REHABILITATION STAFF INVOLVED IN ROLE DEVELOPMENT IMPLEMENTATION

Eighteen staff participated in the implementation of Role Development. Age for these staff ranged from 30 to 55 with a mean age of 41.6. Of the 18 staff, five of the staff were male (28%) and 13 of the staff were female (72%); eight were Caucasian (44%) and 10 were African-American (56%). Staff represented all of the areas within the rehabilitation department. The majority of staff (N = 10; 55%) worked in Recreation, followed by four (22%) in Occupational Therapy, two (11%) in Education, and one each in Vocational Rehabilitation (6%) and Creative Arts (6%). The highest level of education ranged from a High School diploma (50%) to an Associate's Degree (22%), a Bachelor's degree (22%), and a Master's Degree (6%). Eleven staff (61%) were considered to be at the paraprofessional level and seven (39%) were considered to be at the professional level.

All of these staff were required to complete initial assessments and treatment plans, weekly interviews and progress reports, and attend a weekly meeting on the patients in the study. The assessments, treatment plan format, interview, and progress note format were specifically de-

[Haworth co-indexing entry note]: "Response of the Rehabilitation Staff to Role Development." Schindler, Victoria P. Co-published simultaneously in *Occupational Therapy in Mental Health* (The Haworth Press, Inc.) Vol. 20, No. 3/4, 2004, pp. 123-132; and: *Occupational Therapy in Forensic Psychiatry: Role Development and Schizophrenia* (Victoria P. Schindler) The Haworth Press, Inc., 2004, pp. 123-132. Single or multiple copies of this article are available for a fee from The Haworth Document Delivery Service [1-800-HAWORTH, 9:00 a.m. - 5:00 p.m. (EST). E-mail address: docdelivery@haworthpress.com].

http://www.haworthpress.com/web/OTMH
Digital Object Identifier: 10.1300/J004v20n03_09

signed for the study and were distributed as part of the staff training manual. Demographics for the staff involved in Role Development are in Table 28.

At the completion of the study, data were analyzed regarding compliance with the weekly meetings, compliance with the required paperwork, and staff fidelity to the intervention (see Table 28). Level of compliance in attending weekly meetings ranged from 80-100% with a mean of 85% and a mode of 90%. Compliance in completion of required paperwork (i.e., initial assessments, treatment plans, and weekly progress reports) ranged from 0 to 100% with a mean of 77%, median of 83% and a mode of 100%. Fidelity to the intervention was measured via

TABLE 28. Demographic Data for Staff Involved in Role Development Program

Demographic Variable	Total N = 18	%
Age		
30 - 39	8	44.4
40 - 49	6	33.4
50 - 52	4	22.2
Education		
High School Diploma	9	50.0
Associate's Degree	4	22.2
Bachelor's Degree	4	22.2
Master's Degree	1	5.6
Ethnicity		
Caucasian	8	44.4
African American	10	55.6
Gender		
Male	5	27.8
Female	13	72.2
Professional Status		
Professional	7	38.9
Paraprofessional	11	61.1
Department		
Occupational Therapy	4	22.2
Art Therapy	1	5.6
Recreation	10	55.6
Vocational Rehab	1	5.6
Education	2	11.1

two checklists. At least once every two weeks the Principal Investigator visited each staff member in their group and observed the staff providing the intervention to a participant in the study. Based on this observation the Principal Investigator completed a Fidelity Checklist-Principal Investigator of the staff member, and the staff member completed a Fidelity Checklist-Staff Member, on himself/herself.

Compliance on the Fidelity Checklist-Principal Investigator ranged from 50-100% with a mean of 86%, median of 85%, and mode of 80%. Compliance on the Fidelity Checklist-Staff Member ranged from 80-100% with a mean of 86%, median of 100%, and mode of 100% (see Table 29).

Bivariate correlation coefficients were conducted to determine if a relationship existed between the fidelity scores recorded by the Principal Investigator with (1) the fidelity scores recorded by the staff; (2) the

TABLE 29. Compliance Data for Staff Involved in Role Development (N = 18)

Compliance Variable	N	%	Mean	SD
Fidelity - PI Rated			86.4	12
50%	1	5.6		
80 - 89%	10	55.5		
90 - 99%	3	16.7		
100%	4	22.2		
Fidelity - Staff Rated			86.3	31
Did not submit	2	11.1		
80 - 89%	2	11.1		
90 - 99%	4	22.3		
100%	10	55.6		
Paperwork Compliance			76.5	27
Did not submit	2	5.6		
25%	1	5.6		
50%	2	11.1		
75%	1	5.6		
80 - 89%	6	33.3		
90 - 99%	2	11.2		
100%	5	27.8		
Meeting Compliance			85.0	22
80 - 89%	6	33.3		
90 - 99%	8	34.5		
100%	4	27.8		

level of staff compliance with the paperwork (i.e., treatment plans and progress reports); and (3) staff attendance at weekly meetings. A statistically significant correlation existed between Fidelity Checklist-Principal Investigator and Fidelity Checklist-Staff Member (.58, p = .01), and Fidelity Checklist-Principal Investigator and paperwork compliance (.57, p = .01). However, a statistically significant correlation was not achieved between Fidelity Checklist-Principal Investigator and attendance at meetings ($-.07$, p = .77) (see Table 30). This suggests that the Principal Investigator and staff had similar ratings on the Fidelity Checklists and that staff completion of paperwork was related to their level of fidelity to the intervention. It also suggests that a relationship did not exist between fidelity scores recorded by the Principal Investigator and staff attendance at meetings. It should be noted that over the course of the experimental phase of the study, staff absences at the meetings occurred secondary to illness, vacation, and excused absences.

Rehabilitation Staff Focus Groups

As described in Chapter 5, prior to staff training, the Principal Investigator met with 24 rehabilitation staff in pre-training focus groups. Upon completion of the study, the Principal Investigator met with 22 rehabilitation staff in post-study focus groups (one occupational therapy staff member and one art therapist did not have any patients involved in Role Development and therefore did not participate in the post-study focus group). The focus groups were recorded and transcribed. Five to seven questions were addressed in each focus group.

Pre-Training Staff Focus Groups

Five questions were addressed during the pre-training staff focus groups. Staff were given a handout with these questions prior to the start of the focus group. The questions are as follows:

TABLE 30. Bivariate Correlation Coefficients – Staff Fidelity

Variable	Fidelity - Self	Paperwork	Meetings
Fidelity - PI	.58, p = .01	.57, p = .01	$-.07$, p = .77

1. How does your program help the patients to get better?
2. How do you know the patients are getting better? Give examples.
3. What could you do differently to help the patients get better?
4. Do you think you collaborate (work together with the patients)? How?
5. What are some examples of the way you collaborate with the patients?

In response to the first question, five categories of response emerged. Fourteen staff (64%) indicated that their program gives the patient a routine and "something to do." Ten staff (45%) indicated that their program helps the patient increase his social interaction. Nine staff (41%) believed that their program teaches the patient skills such as frustration tolerance or coping skills. Four staff (18%) indicated that their program leads to symptom reduction, and three staff (14%) stated that their program provides education and training to the patients. In commenting on these questions, some staff made statements that seemed to combine categories. One staff member stated, my program " relieves tension and stress and helps the patients take their minds off of other things." Another staff member stated that the programs "relieve tension and frustration and teach the patients how to deal with frustration." Both of these statements appear to address symptom reduction as well as providing the patient with a routine and teaching them skills.

In response to the question, how do you know the patients are getting better, three categories emerged. Twelve staff (55%) cited symptom reduction as an indication that patients are getting better. For example, one staff member stated that patients "are sleeping less and are more alert in their groups." Twelve staff (55%) also described more positive behavior as an indication that patients are improving. One of these staff members stated that patients "have fewer incidents, are more cooperative, and show an increase in their self-control." Eight staff members (36%) stated that they see an improvement in social interaction.

In response to the question, what could you do differently to help the patients get better, six staff (27%) stated that they could provide more compassion and individual attention to the patients. For example, one staff member stated, "I could spend more time with my patients," while another staff stated, "I could find out more about the interests of my patients." Eight staff (36%) spoke of making indirect changes that would affect the environment, the overall schedule, or staff resources or supplies available for group sessions. "I could insure coverage for the evenings or weekends" was a reply offered by one supervisor.

The last two questions addressed the staff's level of collaboration with the patients. Staff were asked how they collaborate with the patients and were asked to provide examples. Twelve staff (55%) described collaboration as a way in which they meet the basic human needs or mental health needs of the patients. Several of these staff stated that they collaborate with their patients by listening to them or establishing a rapport with them. One staff stated, "if the patient is too tired from the medication, I ask him if he has talked with the doctor." A female staff stated, "If there is a home issue or problem, a legal issue, a general health needs, I affirm their concern and treat them as human beings." Eight staff (36%) described collaboration as a way in which they provide education, instruction, or relate expectations to the patients. One of these staff members commented, "I orient them to school, the rehab programs, and the ward issues." Four of the female staff described ways in which they feel that they "provide mothering" to the patients. The female staff described ways that they listen and provide guidance and support and "take care" of the patients by giving them snacks and "a pat on the back."

Several themes consistently emerged through the pre-training focus group questions. It seems apparent that the staff view their involvement with the patients primarily as a means to reduce symptoms, promote positive behaviors, and keep the patients occupied. Although some staff address the learning of skills, this is not a predominant theme. Staff view of collaboration seems to focus more on a style of interacting with the patient rather than working together to identify and address the patients' needs and goals. Although staff interactions with patients seem to be supportive, they seem to be lacking in a few areas. First, staff do not describe an individualized approach that addresses each patient's unique strengths, needs, and situation. Also, they do not describe a method of intervention that focuses on the development of roles and skills.

Post-Study Staff Focus Groups

Seven questions were addressed during the post-study staff focus groups. Staff were given a handout with these questions prior to the start of the focus group. The questions are as follows:

1. Describe the intervention you have been using.
2. Do you think the training has influenced the skills you have to successfully provide treatment to the patients? Which skills?

3. Do you think the training has influenced your ability to help the patients improve? How?
4. Do you think the training has influenced the way you collaborate with your patients? How?
5. Please give an example of how this training has influenced your work with the patients.
6. Do you think the intervention has influenced the patients' treatment–especially their progress or lack of progress? How? Please give some examples of the patients' reactions to the intervention.
7. Do you think the training has had an impact on your job satisfaction?

The first statement required the staff to describe the intervention (i.e., Role Development) they have been using. Three categories of response emerged.

Twelve staff (60%) described it as a method to get to know their patients better or to increase communication with their patients. Seven staff (35%) described it as a method to assess their patients' strengths and limitations and to provide intervention, and seven staff (35%) described it as a method to help patients know their roles.

Questions two and three addressed the effect of the training on staff skills and patient improvement. Because both of these questions addressed the effectiveness of the training, responses were similar and were merged. An overriding theme, cited by at least 55% of the staff, was that the training helped them to view the patient and communicate with him as an "individual" with unique interests and needs. One of these staff members stated, "It helped me to open up and talk with the patients." Fourteen staff (50%) stated that they are now more aware of what they are doing and achieving with their patients, and as a result, they are better able to articulate and document the assessment and intervention process. One staff member stated, "It helped me to articulate why we are doing what we are doing." Six staff (30%) stated it helped them to improve the quality and quantity of their communication with other staff regarding patients' treatment, and five staff (25%) stated that they acquired new methods of intervention and activities to help the patients achieve their roles. One summary statement offered by a supervisor in response to these questions was, "Not only do the patients get enjoyment from participating in their groups, but they get additional help from the staff. Things that they get from here will continue from here."

In response to the fourth question, three categories emerged to address staff collaboration with the patients. Fourteen staff (70%) indicated that the training helped them to give the patients more individualized, personalized attention. Four staff (20%) each indicated that it increased their awareness of the ways that they interact with the patients and that it increases the skills in their intervention with the patients. One of these staff members described how her level of collaboration developed with a patient as follows:

> With Mr. P, when he came into the classroom, he was very quiet. When I sat down with him, he really started opening up to me, what he wants to do here, and what he wants to do when he leaves here, and I really got close to him. So, it helps us to identify and focus on those who are the quiet ones and try to talk to them and bring them out.

Three categories emerged when staff gave examples of how the training influenced their work with the patients. Six staff (30%) cited the example that the training helped them develop a more personal, individualized relationship with the patient. One of these staff members said, "It caused me to set up individual meetings with patients to help them choose individual activities." "With GW, I got to know him and he disclosed he had a drug problem and a desire to be drug-free. He chose the AA slogan 'An attitude of gratitude' and painted it. I hung it on the door and he beamed." Five staff (25%) stated that it helped them to assess the patients' strengths and deficits so they can help them develop a role. One of these staff members stated, "It helped me to help Stephen find a friend." Five staff (25%) described an increase in their communication with other staff regarding patients. For example, one supervisor stated, "I see the staff talking to each other more and that helps you work better with the patients."

When asked if the intervention influenced the patients' treatment, all staff (100%) indicated that it positively influenced their patients' progress. One staff member described the way in which the intervention influenced treatment with one of her patients:

> Today he said he was a little tired with the med changes and so on, but he was now willing to and expressed the language where he would tell me, and we talked, and I don't know if that would have happened if the whole process weren't in place. I mean, he is generally a quiet man, and wants to get lost and keep things very quiet

and to himself, but he really did express his needs in a very appropriate way, and we worked through it. We worked out a compromise and it helped him to focus on his role here and to keep working as opposed to sleeping or goofing off or whatever other options he would have come up with. He generally worked everyday and was very persistent even though the skills are still slow to develop. He had incredible self-motivation and continues to have it. I think that overall it was very positive.

Additionally, nine staff (45%) indicated that patients' communication increases when staff take a more individualized, personalized approach with them. One of these staff members described progress she observed over time as she increased her level of communication with one of the patients:

> Matthew–at first he would not look at you, gave you no eye contact, when you talked to him, he would just shake his head as you talked with him, and at the end he came running up to me and said, "Hey, Phyllis, I have to talk to you." He almost scared me. He really flourished at the end.

Three staff (15%) stated the intervention gave them more options for assessment and intervention with the patients. For example, one staff member stated, "Regarding G's role as a student, it allowed us to focus on that in terms of 'I am a student and this is how a student is expected to act and react and so on.' I see this as positive."

In the final question, staff were asked if the training had an impact on their job satisfaction. Four categories emerged. Eight staff (40%) stated they feel more capable, seven staff (35%) stated it gave them a new skill, and two staff (10%) stated they feel happier and more fulfilled. One staff member commented, "It improves your competencies and self-esteem regarding your abilities as a group leader in providing assessment and evaluation of patients." Another staff member stated, "I don't care if she (i.e., the Principal Investigator) gives me 10 patients, it's a great learning experience." However, three staff (15%) cited that it is "more work." One staff member stated, "The weekly interviews and progress reports were too much to keep up with–especially if you have three or four patients in the study at the same time."

Three themes that consistently emerged throughout the post-study focus groups were: (1) the intervention provided a means to develop a more individualized, personalized relationship with the patient; (2) the intervention helped staff increase their repertoire of skills for assessment and intervention; and (3) the intervention helped staff to be more aware of and articulate their interaction and intervention with the patient. Additionally, in comparison to the pre-training focus groups, staff were able to provide a more accurate description of "collaboration" with the patient and to describe a method in which they interacted with the patient as an unique individual, and helped the patient identify and develop skills and roles that are meaningful to him.

CONCLUSION

Demographic data on the staff described a primarily female, paraprofessional staff with overall good compliance to the training and intervention involved with the Role Development program. Through pre-training and post-study focus groups, staff were able to identify meaningful ways in which they used Role Development to help participants develop skills and roles, and in which Role Development enhanced their skills.

Chapter 10

An Analysis of the Effectiveness
of the Intervention

INTRODUCTION

There were several important findings in this study. First, there was statistically significant improvement in task skills, interpersonal skills, and role functioning among participants involved in the Role Development program, especially at four weeks of treatment. In contrast, participants involved in the comparison group, the multidepartmental activity program, showed less improvement, no improvement, or an actual decrease in their task and interpersonal skills. Furthermore, participants in the Role Development program were able to describe the positive changes they experienced as well as long-term benefits as a result of their participation in the program. Although the participants in the multidepartmental activity program described some positive attributes of their program, they could not describe any specific benefits or long-term benefits of that program. Support for the Role Development program was also evident in the feedback from the staff who participated in the training and implementation of the program. Upon completion of the study, staff described the intervention as a means to develop a more personalized, collaborative relationship with their patients as well as a means to increase staff skills.

[Haworth co-indexing entry note]: "An Analysis of the Effectiveness of the Intervention." Schindler, Victoria P. Co-published simultaneously in *Occupational Therapy in Mental Health* (The Haworth Press, Inc.) Vol. 20, No. 3/4, 2004, pp. 133-149; and: *Occupational Therapy in Forensic Psychiatry: Role Development and Schizophrenia* (Victoria P. Schindler) The Haworth Press, Inc., 2004, pp. 133-149. Single or multiple copies of this article are available for a fee from The Haworth Document Delivery Service [1-800-HAWORTH, 9:00 a.m. - 5:00 p.m. (EST). E-mail address: docdelivery@haworthpress.com].

http://www.haworthpress.com/web/OTMH
Digital Object Identifier: 10.1300/J004v20n03_10

The discussion will address each of the above findings in accordance with the research hypotheses. Implications for the study will be described. Limitations to the study will be presented and the chapter will finish with a conclusion.

IMPROVEMENT IN TASK SKILLS BETWEEN THE COMPARISON AND EXPERIMENTAL GROUPS

The first hypothesis stated that participants involved in the Role Development program would demonstrate greater improvement in task skills in comparison to participants in the multidepartmental activity program. Results of the study demonstrated statistically significant findings. Analysis of the within-group tests, ANCOVA, repeated measures ANOVA, MANCOVA, and the qualitative findings all supported this hypothesis.

Within-group tests showed that participants in the Role Development program demonstrated statistically significant improvement in task skills at the four and eight week posttest. Although these participants did not demonstrate statistically significant differences in task skills at the 12-week posttest, they did show an increase in mean scores indicating that they were able to maintain or slightly increase their level of task skills. In contrast, participants in the multidepartmental activity program did not demonstrate statistically significant improvement at any of the posttests. In fact, mean scores decreased from the pretest to the four-week posttest indicating a decrease in task skills. Although mean scores increased at the eight and 12-week posttests, the increase in scores was small, indicating a slight but nonsignificant level of improvement in task skills.

Results of the ANCOVA also demonstrated statistically significant findings, which further strengthens the difference in the development of task skills between the two groups. Because the ANCOVA maximizes the capacity to detect differences (Burns & Grove, 1993), this test provided strong support for the difference in improvement of task skills between the two groups. Repeated measures ANOVA demonstrated statistically significant within-group and between-group findings. The MANCOVA assessed the effect of the Role Development program on a combined dependent variable (Task Skills Scale, Interpersonal Skills Scale, and the Role Functioning Scale). The Task Skills Scale represents one part of the combined dependent variable. Results of this test demonstrated statistically significant findings lending additional support to the improvement in task skills in the group participating in the Role Development program.

Further support for these findings emerged from the qualitative data. Although participants in the comparison group felt as though the multi-departmental activity program was helpful to the extent that it provided a means to occupy their time, they did not feel as though they learned skills necessary for their current recovery or for long-term benefit. In contrast, the participants in the Role Development program were specifically able to identify task skills as skills they learned, such as their ability to focus on and successfully complete their work. Additionally, they were able to describe these skills as uniquely addressing their needs and providing a link to skills they will need in their future life situations.

IMPROVEMENT IN INTERPERSONAL SKILLS BETWEEN THE COMPARISON AND EXPERIMENTAL GROUPS

The second hypothesis stated that participants involved in the Role Development program would demonstrate greater improvement in interpersonal skills in comparison to participants in the multidepartmental activity program. Results of the study demonstrated statistically significant findings. Analysis of the within-group tests, ANCOVA, repeated measures ANOVA, MANCOVA, and the qualitative findings all support this hypothesis.

Within-group tests showed that participants in the Role Development program demonstrated statistically significant improvement in interpersonal skills at the four-week posttest. Although participants in this program did not demonstrate statistically significant differences at the eight and 12 week posttests, the mean change scores (8 week, +1.88 mean change; 12 week, +.73 mean change) showed improvement at both of these posttests. This may indicate that although these participants did not continue to demonstrate levels of positive change, they maintained or slightly improved their increased level of interpersonal skills, especially at eight weeks of treatment. In contrast, participants in the multidepartmental activity program did not demonstrate statistically significant improvement at any of the posttests. Although mean score changes demonstrated slight improvement at the eight week posttest (+.7 mean change; p = .427), this was followed by a decline in scores at the 12 week posttest (+.1 mean change; p = .821), indicating that if there was an improvement in skills, it was short-lived.

As seen with task skills, results of the ANCOVA also demonstrated statistically significant findings, further indicating the development of interpersonal skills between the two groups. Because the ANCOVA maximizes the capacity to detect differences (Burns & Grove, 1993), this test provides strong evidence that there was a difference in improvement of interpersonal skills between the two groups. Repeated measures ANOVA demonstrated statistically significant within-group and between-group findings. As described in the previous section, the MANCOVA assessed the effect of the Role Development program on a combined variable of the three scales. Results of this test demonstrated statistically significant findings lending additional support to the improvement in interpersonal skills in the group participating in the Role Development program.

As found in the previous discussion on task skills, further support from these findings emerged from the qualitative data. Almost all group treatment activities leading to the development of roles require a combination of task and interpersonal skills. Whereas participants in the comparison group were unable to identify skills they learned either for immediate or long-term use, participants in the Role Development program were specifically able to identify interpersonal skills as skills they learned. As with task skills, these participants were also able to see the interpersonal skills as uniquely addressing their needs and providing a link to skills they will need in their future life situations.

DEVELOPMENT OF SOCIAL ROLES BETWEEN THE COMPARISON AND EXPERIMENTAL GROUPS

The third hypothesis stated that participants involved in the Role Development program would develop more social roles in comparison to participants in the multidepartmental activity program. The Role Functioning Scale and the Role Checklist were used as indicators of social role development. Results of between-group tests, within-group tests, repeated measures ANOVA on the Role Functioning Scale, the MANCOVA and the qualitative findings demonstrated results that support the hypothesis.

Between-group tests of the Role Functioning Scale showed that participants in the experimental group demonstrated greater improvement in social role functioning than participants in the comparison group at the four-week posttest, but not at the eight week or 12 week posttests. Within-group tests indicated that the experimental group demonstrated statistically significant improvement at all three posttests. In contrast, within-group tests indicated that the comparison group demonstrated statistically significant improvement at the four-week posttest but not at the eight week or 12 week posttests. Closer examination of these findings at the four-week posttest indicated that participants in the experimental group demonstrated a greater degree of change in each of the four roles in the Role Functioning Scale. Repeated measures ANOVA demonstrated statistically significant within-group and between-group findings. Results of the MANCOVA demonstrated statistically significant findings lending additional support to the improvement in role functioning in the group participating in the Role Development program.

As found in the previous discussion on task and interpersonal skills, further support from these findings emerged from the qualitative data. Whereas participants in the comparison group were unable to identify roles they learned either for immediate or long-term use, participants in the Role Development program were able to identify specific roles they developed and how these roles would be useful to them in their future life situations.

Although results from the Role Checklist did add interesting, useful data to the overall findings, this instrument could not be used in the way it was originally intended. A detailed explanation of this can be found in Chapter 6. The quantitative findings did not directly address the hypothesis. Nevertheless, it was interesting to learn that despite the fact that the patients involved in the study have severe and persistent mental illness, long psychiatric history, criminal charges, and low levels of education, at least one-half of the patients identified each role as a role he would like to have in the future. This demonstrates a desire and willingness to begin or resume a typical life. This is often the first step toward rehabilitation (Hocking, 2001; Stuve & Menditto, 1999).

Additional interesting findings from the Role Checklist were the correlations between past, current, and future roles for the two groups of participants. Patients in the experimental group may have had a greater number of statistically significant correlations between these time frames because they knew they would be encouraged and assisted to develop these roles.

RELATIONSHIP OF TIME TO THE DEVELOPMENT OF TASK SKILLS, INTERPERSONAL SKILLS, AND SOCIAL ROLES

The final hypothesis stated that the longer an individual is involved in the Role Development program, the greater the effect on the development of task skills, interpersonal skills and social roles. Several of the statistical tests supported this hypothesis. Within-group tests on the Task Skills Scale, Interpersonal Skills Scale, and Role Functioning Scale all measured change over time. All of these tests showed statistically significant change in the experimental group at four weeks of treatment. However, results of these tests varied at eight and 12 weeks of treatment for the experimental group. Within-group tests of the Task Skills Scale demonstrated statistically significant change at eight weeks, but not at 12 weeks of treatment whereas within-group tests of the Interpersonal Skills Scale did not demonstrate statistically significant change at eight or 12 weeks. Within-group tests of the Role Functioning Scale demonstrated statistically significant change at eight and 12 weeks of treatment. Although there was a lack of change at certain points in time, participants may have maintained previous progress that was made.

In addition to the findings of the above tests, repeated measures analysis of variance was conducted independently with each of the three scales. This statistical measure examines multiple observations of a scale over time and/or under different conditions and is considered a stronger measure of change over time than within-group tests conducted between posttests on each individual scale (Green et al., 2000). Repeated measures ANOVA was used to assess between-group differences and within-group differences over time. Statistically significant findings were found with p values ranging from .028 to .000 among the three scales. These findings demonstrated that not only did the participants in the experimental group show an improvement in their skills and roles over time, but that their improvement was also greater than the participants in the comparison group.

Results of the qualitative findings further support this hypothesis. Only participants who completed the entire 12 weeks in either study were interviewed. As has been indicated earlier, only participants in the experimental group were able to cite specific skills and roles they learned through participation in the program and ways in which these skills and roles could transfer to other life situations. Although staff in the focus groups were not specifically asked about differences in changes over time between the two methods of treatment, themes that emerged from the qualitative staff findings do suggest that the Role Development program would continue to be effective and meaningful over time. For example, staff consistently stated that the intervention based on the Role Development program provided a means to develop a more personalized, collaborative relationship with their patients. It would follow that the longer a staff member is in a therapeutic relationship with a patient, the more personalized and collaborative the relationship would become and the more the patient will improve.

IMPLICATIONS OF THE STUDY

There are important implications of this study. First, individuals diagnosed with a severe and persistent mental illness, such as one of the schizophrenic disorders, are both willing and able to develop roles and the skills that are the foundation to these roles. Also, these individuals are able to identify specific roles they would like to develop and how these roles may be useful to them in their future life situations. Secondly, rehabilitation staff, including paraprofessional staff, are willing and able to successfully learn and implement a theory-based intervention that ultimately helps their patients.

Implications for the Client Population

Individuals diagnosed with schizophrenic disorders, especially those committed to a maximum-security facility, are not often offered comprehensive rehabilitation treatment. Comprehensive treatment, if offered at all, is usually reserved for clients in the community or transitioning to the community. Perhaps the rationale is that the individuals who are institutionalized are not capable of or motivated toward participating in comprehensive treatment leading to self-improvement and productive participation in society. However, this study demonstrates that individuals living with multiple disabling factors, such as a long psychiatric history, legal charges, and low levels of education, can develop skills and roles in as little as four weeks. Stuve and Menditto (1999) advocated that all individuals diagnosed with mental illness are "rehabilitation-ready" (p. 36) regardless of the setting in which the person resides, if the appropriate rehabilitation treatment is provided. Anthony Lehman (1999), who directed the Patient Outcomes Research Team (PORT) project for the Agency for Health Care Policy and Research (AHCPR) and the National Institute for Mental Health (NIMH) (1988), also strongly advocated for rehabilitation treatment for all individuals diagnosed with schizophrenia. He has often cited the necessity of simultaneous pharmacoptherapy and psychosocial treatments. He states that rehabilitation is most important when an individual is stable on medication but still living with the symptoms of a persistent mental illness. This accurately describes the scenario for the participants in this study.

The improvement of the participants in the Role Development program demonstrates that despite complicating life factors and residual effects of a severe mental illness, individuals recently stabilized on medication are willing and able to develop skills and meaningful roles. A discussion of the "Top 10 Health Challenges" (Fleming & Kaplan, 2000, p. 1698) of the 21st century also stressed the need for effective treatment for individuals with serious mental illness. These health challenges, which were identified by the Centers for Disease Control (CDC) and published in the Journal of the American Medical Association, cited mental illness as the second leading cause of disability and premature mortality in the U.S., and urged researchers to improve access to treatment and promote good mental health. The Role Development program provides treatment and promotes improvement in mental health to a mentally ill population in a maximum-security psychiatric setting.

ATTRIBUTES OF THE ROLE DEVELOPMENT PROGRAM THAT PROMOTE CLIENT SUCCESS

The success of the Role Development program leads to the question: what are the attributes of this program that contribute to the improvement of individuals who participated in it? The Role Development program has a number of different attributes that may have contributed to successful outcomes. First, the intervention is based on a theoretical set of guidelines for practice, is a collaborative and client-centered approach, and focuses on evaluation and treatment of meaningful occupation. Each attribute may contribute to successful treatment, but it may be the combination of attributes that is the formula for success. The result is that the Role Development program can promote an increased quality of life in individuals diagnosed with schizophrenia.

Set of Guidelines for Practice

Interventions based on a set of guidelines for practice contain a theoretical foundation that is linked to evaluation and principles to promote change. The theoretical base is developed from a comprehensive review of the literature and provides a foundation for treatment. Evaluation and treatment principles are derived from this base. This promotes a logical and consistent course of action. Although it is the process derived from the practice guidelines that is being tested, and not the theoretical base, the theoretical foundation is necessary to develop an effective intervention (Mosey, 1986, 1996). Role Development is based on a strong theoretical foundation and all the requisite evaluation and treatment components of effective practice guidelines.

Collaborative, Client-Centered Approach

Role Development is also a collaborative, client-centered approach to treatment. Mattingly and Fleming (1994) describe collaboration as a clinical reasoning process that engages the patient in many choices and decisions regarding evaluation and treatment. It describes a process in which the clinician makes an effort to get to know the patient as a "person"–his/her roles, interests, social and cultural background–so that choices in therapy can be geared to specific needs. Client-centered practice has been defined as "an approach to service which embraces a philosophy of respect for, and partnership with, people receiving services" (Law, Baptiste, & Mills, 1995, p. 253). A client-centered model of practice includes components such as flexible, individualized service delivery, facilitation of client participation in all aspects of treatment, and information and emotional support (Law & Mills, 1998, p. 9). Law (1998) states that patients who feel they have been respected and treated as a partner in their treatment are more satisfied with and successful in their treatment, and she provides multiple examples of studies supporting this hypothesis. She also states that despite all of the positive outcomes of client-centered practice, many practitioners do not practice from this perspective because it can be time-consuming and challenging. Nevertheless, Role Development incorporates many of the concepts of collaborative, client-centered practice.

From the start of the intervention, the participants choose the roles that are meaningful to them and that they would like to develop. The activities and social situations to develop the roles and skills are selected in partnership with the participant, and weekly interviews are conducted to assess the participant's perception of progress. There is ongoing, personal interaction between the client and the staff member. This process occurs in a continuous cycle throughout participation in the Role Development program. The qualitative findings attest to the importance of this aspect of the program. The staff felt a sense of satisfaction in developing a more individualized, personalized relationship with the participant and the patients in the Role Development program were able to identify skills and roles that met their personal needs and situations.

An additional finding of the study that supports the use of a collaborative, client-centered approach involves the subgroup of patients who received individual attention as part of their involvement in the multi-departmental activity program. It is interesting to note that this sub-group did not show any statistically significant difference in scores on any of the scales in comparison to the subgroup that did not receive individual attention. This attests to the finding that attention alone will not lead to improvement in task skills, interpersonal skills, or role functioning. It is the nature and quality of the attention that promotes improvement. Because the Role Development program is based on a theoretical set of guidelines for practice, attention provided through this program was specifically structured to include personalized, respectful discussions that addressed the participant's needs, goals, and progress.

Focus on Meaningful Occupation

Role Development also focuses on evaluation and treatment of meaningful occupation. Although many writers throughout the 20th century, especially in occupational therapy, have insisted that therapy be provided in a context of meaningful occupation (Clark, 1997; Fidler, 1969; Reilly, 1962; Slagle, 1924), some writers have also directed our attention to examples of treatment practices that continue to occur despite being meaningless, irrelevant, repetitive and condescending to the client (Crabtree, 1998; Law & Mills, 1998; Mattingly & Fleming, 1994). Evaluation and treatment that focus on the components of occupations without focusing on the occupation as a whole, are often viewed as boring and irrelevant to the person receiving the service (Hocking, 2001). For example, engaging a client in an activity to improve task skills without linking the activity and skills to a role or occupation will create confusion and dissatisfaction with the intervention. Role Development, with its premise of building skills within the context of roles that are meaningful to the client, promotes the building of significant improvements in the quantitative measures as well as in the statements of the qualitative findings. The patients in the Role Development program were not only able to identify skills and roles they learned, but were also able to describe specific ways in which the skills and roles could generalize to other life situations. The patients in the multidepartmental activity program did not make the same claims about their treatment program. Perhaps this difference occurred because the multidepartmental activity program focused on the productive use of time and the learning of skills in isolation from meaningful roles or occupation. In addition, the staff involved in the Role Development program cited an increase in their repertoire of skills for assessment and intervention within their role of clinician or group leader. As a result, it can be noted that transfer of learning occurred among staff developing broader and deeper professional roles.

Promoting Quality of Life

The link between rehabilitation and improving quality of life is an important link that is achieved through the Role Development program. Sartoris (1992) outlined five characteristics of a rehabilitation program that successfully promotes quality of life: (1) improvement in quality of life as a result of participation in a rehabilitation program must be perceived by patients and their families; (2) rehabilitation should not be done *for* people but *with* them; (3) people are different and rehabilitation programs should reflect differing needs; (4) disabled people and their impairments change over time and rehabilitation programs must adapt according to these changes; and (5) rehabilitation services and other services aiming to help people in other ways need to be meshed (p. 1181). The Role Development program addresses each of these characteristics. It advocates an individualized, collaborative approach and the constant active involvement of the patient outlined in the first four characteristics.

The attributes of the Role Development program contributing to improved quality of life can be linked to factors identified as important by persons diagnosed with schizophrenia. Labierte-Rudman, Yu, Scott, and Pajouhandeh (2000) conducted focus groups with 35 individuals diagnosed with schizophrenia to determine factors important to quality of life. Themes emerging from these groups focused on managing time, connecting and belonging, and making choices and maintaining control. These themes exemplify basic needs with which we can all identify, regardless of our state of ability or disability. Each of these themes can be linked to an aspect of the Role Development program. Within the theme of managing time, the individuals in the focus groups stated that they want to use their time in the same way most people do–involved in roles and activities and interactions that are productive, meaningful and balanced. The quantitative and qualitative results of the Role Development program overwhelmingly support the development of roles and skills that are personal and meaningful. Within the theme of connecting and belonging, the importance of relationships emerges. The Role Development program not only fosters staff/patient relationships, but also helps the patient to develop roles involving relationships and the interpersonal skills that lead to success in these roles. Lastly, the theme of making choices and maintaining control points to the need for a sense of independence and control over decisions in one's life. The collaborative, client-centered approach of the Role Development program recognizes the importance of this need.

The Role Development program is not a complex, complicated or difficult intervention. It is based on some very simple, common principles of collaboration and meaningfulness. Results of this study demonstrate that in as few as four weeks of treatment, individuals with severe mental illness can show improvement in task and interpersonal skills and social roles. Additionally, comments from both the staff and patients indicate that this is a meaningful treatment approach that not only promotes patient success but also provides additional job satisfaction. Used in collaboration with other multidisciplinary treatment approaches, it is effective in promoting positive change and improved quality of life for individuals diagnosed with schizophrenia.

IMPLICATIONS OF THE STUDY

Implications for Rehabilitation Staff

Another important finding of this study is that rehabilitation staff, especially paraprofessional staff, are capable of successfully learning and implementing a theory-based intervention that ultimately helps their patients.

The staff involved in the Role Development program were primarily early middle-aged, female, paraprofessional staff. Prior to the training in Role Development, the staff identified traits such as kindness and helpfulness as traits supporting client improvement, but characteristics needed for a successful rehabilitation program, such as the development of individualized, flexible rehabilitation approaches (Sartorius, 1992), were not identified. Stuve and Menditto (1999) claimed that patients with severe mental illness benefit from appropriate rehabilitation treatment. They also proposed that staff working in state hospitals can provide effective rehabilitation treatment if they participate in appropriate training. They recommended incorporating several components into such a training program, and these were used in the training in Role Development. For example, the authors state that staff typically do for patients rather than with patients. Sartorius (1992) cited this same dilemma. Stuve and Menditto (1992) recommended a shift in thinking to counteract this widely-held practice. The collaborative, client-centered approach used in Role Development accomplishes this shift in thinking. The authors also recommended that staff receive training in developing and implementing normalizing experiences for their patients. The patient's selection of personal, meaningful roles, and the activities and interactions to develop these roles within the Role Development program, is an example of a normalizing activity.

Corrigan and McCracken (1995) also proposed a shift in the way training is conducted for psychiatric rehabilitation staff. They stated that typical rehabilitation training involves off-site training that rarely translates into practice when the staff return to their work settings. The authors called for a paradigm shift in training and recommend several training techniques. For example, the authors recommended user-friendly training programs, interactive staff training, ongoing supervision to implement the new skills learned, and levels of assessment to determine the effectiveness of the training. The authors stressed that the ultimate efficacy of a training program is determined by its effects on the patients. Moncher and Prinz (1991) found that clear written materials, didactic teaching, role-plays, and supervision promote learning and application of the new information. Durlak (1988) found that treatment manuals or comprehensive written materials reduce the variance in treatment administration and guide and standardize the learning and subsequent treatment implementation. The Role Development training program incorporated these recommendations as well as other characteristics to promote successful training and staff fidelity to the training.

The Role Development training program incorporated several methods of teaching. In the course of the 15.5 hours of formal training, lecture, role-playing, and small group work were used as teaching methods. For example, staff developed role-play skits to practice the initial and weekly interviews required between staff and patients. These methods promoted a user-friendly and interactive training program. Individual training in which the Principal Investigator worked with each staff member in his/her work area followed formal training. These methods provided ongoing supervision so the staff could develop a level of competency prior to implementation of the experimental aspect of the study. Fidelity to the training was monitored once the study began. Of course, the ultimate measure of effective training is in the effectiveness of the treatment. The quantitative and qualitative results support patient improvement and the staff comments in the qualitative results attest to this. For example, the staff expressed satisfaction in their ability to develop individualized, personal relationships with the patients and in the improvement in their assessment and intervention skills.

Although the staff were at different levels in terms of years of experience and level of education, each staff member was able to develop improved skills. Professional level staff, already familiar with theory-based interventions, were able to improve the quality of their intervention with the patients whereas paraprofessional staff were able to learn and implement a theory-based intervention.

Administrative Implications

As a result of the study, the administration at the facility in which the study occurred has adopted Role Development as a measure of ongoing clinical competency to meet requirements of the Joint Commission of Accreditation of Hospital Organizations (JCAHO) and Center for Medicaid/Medicare Services (CMS). Individuals diagnosed with schizophrenic disorders who are committed to the facility for treatment and eventual discharge to a less restrictive setting will participate in treatment based on Role Development. Additionally, the administration completed a reorganization of staff supervision so professional staff will clinically supervise paraprofessional staff. Administrative procedures have been developed so that all staff continue to participate in the Role Development program and receive supervision in this process. New staff will be trained by the rehabilitation supervisors.

LIMITATIONS OF THE STUDY

There are several limitations to the study. One limitation concerns the generalizability of the study findings (Burns & Grove, 1993; Portnoy & Watkins, 2000). There is the possibility that the results may not generalize to individuals in other treatment settings such as acute hospital settings or outpatient settings. It is not known if skills and roles can be learned in less than four weeks in other settings and many inpatient treatment settings have a length of stay that is shorter than four weeks. Also, the participants in this study were a "captive audience." Because they were involuntarily committed to the facility, it was guaranteed that they would spend four hours per day in the treatment program. This may not be so in other types of settings, especially outpatient settings. However, the guarantee of participation was also true for the participants in the comparison group, and they did not show the level of improvement evidenced in the participants in the Role Development program.

Some limitations can affect the internal validity of the study. One of these limitations concerns the patient participants. All participants received additional treatment during the course of the study including medication and other interventions from psychology, social work, and nursing. However, it should be noted that every patient in the entire study was prescribed antipsychotic medication. In the facility in which the study occurred, a diagnosis of a schizophrenic disorder warrants intervention with antipsychotic medication. Additionally, all patients receive intervention from psychology, social work, and nursing. Therefore, the effect of other interventions was equalized over both groups.

Another limitation of the study is that staff involved in the Role Development program may not be typical of staff in other treatment settings. Certain characteristics of the staff, such as their age, gender, or years of experience, may make this staff more amenable to training than other staff. Also, certain characteristics of this rehabilitation department may not be typical of rehabilitation departments in other settings. It is the policy of this department to conduct ongoing, competency-based training. Staff in this department are accustomed to this. This may not be true for staff in other rehabilitation departments.

Instrumentation was a limitation for two of the four instruments in this study. Although inter-rater reliability, test-retest reliability, and internal consistency were obtained on the Task Skills Scale and the Interpersonal Skills Scale prior to their use in the study, these instruments were developed for use in this study and other measures of validity and reliability have not been conducted. However, standardized instruments that measure the task and interpersonal skills (as they pertain to this study) were not located despite an extensive review of the literature.

Because the study occurred over the course of 13 months, the historical nature of this design may be a limitation. Participants in the comparison and experimental groups could have differed from each other because these groups were conducted in a consecutive manner. Also, changes other than the treatment interventions, such as changes in staffing due to staff turnover or a substantial change in the setting during the time the study was conducted, could have been responsible for changes in participant behavior (Burns & Grove, 1993; Portnoy & Watkins, 2000). These potential limitations were monitored. There were no statistically significant differences in demographics between the comparison and experimental groups so the samples did not differ from each other. Also, although there were small changes in the treatment setting (e.g., staff illness, vacation), there were no changes in the staff involved in the study (e.g., staff turnover) nor any substantial changes in the setting that would be responsible for differences in participant behavior between the comparison and experimental groups.

IMPLICATIONS FOR FUTURE RESEARCH

Further research is needed to replicate this study among patients and staff in other types of settings. Also, additional questions have emerged that require future study. Participants in this study showed statistically significant change in as few as four weeks of treatment, but in some instances did not continue to show statistically significant levels of change as treatment progressed. Can the development of roles and skills occur in less than four weeks? Do clients achieve a certain level of skills and roles and then plateau? Do they plateau because they need to transfer learning or generalize by way of applying their new skills in the real world? Or do they plateau because they need to expand their Role Development to other roles not applicable or feasible on an inpatient service, such as roles of family member or community member? It would also be interesting to study which types of clients benefit the most from this intervention. As was discovered in an in-depth view of pretest differences, there was a subgroup of participants in the comparison group who scored high (score of 4 on a 5-point scale) on the pretest on the Task Skills Scale and the Interpersonal Skills Scale. Although these participants were not involved in the Role Development program, it would be interesting to study if participants with high pretest scores decline, maintain, or continue to improve their skills and roles over time.

CHAPTER CONCLUSION

This study has demonstrated several statistically significant findings that have important implications for treatment of people diagnosed with mental illness.

Quantitative and qualitative findings support each of the hypotheses. Implications of the study are supported by current literature. Rationale for providing meaningful treatment for this challenging population is provided along with findings supporting the readiness of this population for treatment they perceive as helpful. Rationale supporting the training of state hospital staff, especially paraprofessional staff, in a theory-based treatment intervention is provided and supported. Administrative implications supporting the use of Role Development were also outlined.

Limitations to the study are described. Although there are some important limitations to consider, the overall findings of the study are important for the mental health community. It is very promising and heartening to demonstrate that individuals diagnosed with a severe and persistent mental illness are both willing and able to develop skills and roles. As important, rehabilitation staff, especially paraprofessional staff, are willing and able to successfully learn and implement a theory-based intervention that ultimately helps their patients. It is hoped that the Role Development treatment guidelines for practice can be applied to other settings and populations so that they also may benefit from the challenge and effort to grow psychosocially as people who enjoy being in roles, as both participants and staff did in this study.

References

American Psychiatric Association (2000). *Diagnostic and statistical manual of mental disorders IV-R* (4th ed.). Washington, DC: Author.

American Psychiatric Association (1997). Practice guidelines for the treatment of patients with schizophrenia. Supplement to *American Journal of Psychiatry, 154* (4).

Andrews, G. (1995, May/June). Best practices for implementing outcomes management. *Behavioral Healthcare Tomorrow, 4,* 19-21, 74-75.

Anthony, W. A. (1993). Recovery from mental illness: The guiding vision of the mental health system in the 1990's. *Innovations & Research, 2*(3), 17-24.

Anthony, W. A., & Liberman, R. P. (1986). The practice of psychiatric rehabilitation: Historical, conceptual, and research base. *Schizophrenia Bulletin, 12*(4), 542-559.

Anthony, W. A., & Margules, A. (1974). Toward improving the efficacy of psychiatric rehabilitation: A skills training approach. *Rehabilitation Psychology, 21,* 101-105.

Bandura, A. (1977). *Social learning theory.* Englewood Cliffs, NJ: Prentice-Hall.

Barbour, A., & Moreno, Z. T. (1980). Role fatigue. *Group Psychotherapy, Psychodrama, and Sociometry, 33,* 185-190.

Barker, S., Barron, N., McFarland, B. H., & Bigelow, D. H. (1994). A community ability scale for chronically mentally ill consumers–Reliability and validity. *Community Mental Health Journal, 30* (4), 363-379.

Baronet, A. M., & Gerber, G. J. (1998). Psychiatric rehabilitation: Efficacy of four models. *Clinical Psychology Review, 18,* 189-228.

Barris, R., Dickie, V., & Baron, K. B. (1988). A comparison of psychiatric patients and normal subjects based on the Model of Human Occupation. *Occupational Therapy Journal of Research, 8,* 3-23.

Barris, R., Oakley, F., & Kielhofner, G. (1988). The Role Checklist. In B. Hemphill (Ed.), *Mental health assessment in occupational therapy* (pp. 73-91). Thorofare, NJ: Slack.

Bavaro, S. M. (1991). Occupational therapy and obsessive-compulsive disorder. *American Journal of Occupational Therapy, 45,* 456-458.

[Haworth co-indexing entry note]: "References." Schindler, Victoria P. Co-published simultaneously in *Occupational Therapy in Mental Health* (The Haworth Press, Inc.) Vol. 20, No. 3/4, 2004, pp. 151-159; and: *Occupational Therapy in Forensic Psychiatry: Role Development and Schizophrenia* (Victoria P. Schindler) The Haworth Press, Inc., 2004, pp. 151-159. Single or multiple copies of this article are available for a fee from The Haworth Document Delivery Service [1-800-HAWORTH, 9:00 a.m. - 5:00 p.m. (EST). E-mail address: docdelivery@haworthpress.com].

Digital Object Identifier: 10.1300/J004v20n03_11

Benne, K., & Sheats, P. (1978). Functional roles of group members. In L. Bradford (Ed.), *Group Development* (2nd ed., pp. 52-61). La Jolla, CA: University Associates.

Biddle, B. J. (1979). *Role theory: Expectations, identities, and behaviors.* New York: Academic Press.

Black, M. M. (1976). The occupational career. *American Journal of Occupational Therapy, 30,* 225-228.

Blume, T. W., Green, S., Joanning, H., & Quinn, W. S. (1994). Social role negotiation skills for substance-abusing adolescents: A group model. *Journal of Substance Abuse Treatment, 11* (3), 197-204.

Blumer, H. (1969). *Symbolic interactionism: Perspective and method.* Englewood Cliffs, NJ: Prentice-Hall.

Branholm, I. B., & Fugl-Meyer, A. (1992). Occupational role preferences and life satisfaction. *Occupational Therapy Journal of Research, 12,* 159-171.

Brekke, J. S. (1992). An examination of the relationships among three outcome scales in schizophrenia. *Journal of Nervous and Mental Disease, 180* (3), 162-167.

Brekke, J. S., & Barrio (1997). Cross-ethnic symptom differences in schizophrenia: The influence of culture and minority status. *Schizophrenia Bulletin, 23* (3), 305-316.

Brekke, J. S., Long, J. D., Nesbit, N., & Sobel, E. (1997). The impact of service characteristics on functional outcomes from community support programs for persons with schizophrenia: A growth curve analysis. *Journal of Consulting and Clinical Psychology, 65,* 464-475.

Brekke, J. S., & Mathiesen, S. G. (1995). Effects of parental involvement on the functioning of noninstitutionalized adults with schizophrenia. *Psychiatric Services, 46,* 1149-1155.

Brekke, J. S., Raine, A., Ansel, M., Lencz, T., & Bird, L. (1997). Neuropsychological and psychophysiological correlates of psychosocial functioning in schizophrenia. *Schizophrenia Bulletin, 23* (1), 19-28.

Broekema, M. C., Danz, K. H., & Schloemer, C. U. (1975). *American Journal of Occupational Therapy, 29,* 22-27.

Bruce, B., & Borg, M. A. (1991). *The group system: The therapeutic activity group in occupational therapy.* Thorofare, NJ: Slack

Bruner, J. S. (1966). *Toward a theory of instruction.* Cambridge, MA: Belknap Press.

Burns, N., & Grove, S. K. (1993). *The practice of nursing research: Conduct, critique and utilization* (2nd ed.). Philadelphia: W. B. Saunders.

Callero, P. L. (1994). From role-playing to role-using: Understanding role as resource. *Social Psychology Quarterly, 57,* 228-243.

Campbell, D. T., & Stanley, J. C. (1963). *Experimental and quasi-experimental designs for research.* Chicago: Rand McNally College Publishing.

Cara, E., & MacRae, A. (1998). *Psychosocial occupational therapy: A clinical practice.* Albany, NY: Delmar.

Clark, F., Azen, S. P., Zemke, R., Jackson, J., Carlson, M., Mandel, D., Hay, J., Josephson, K., Cherry, B., Hessel, C., Palmer, J., & Lipson, L. (1997). Occupational therapy for independent-living older adults. *Journal of the American Medical Association, 278,* 1321-1326.

Cohen, J. (1988). *Statistical power analysis for the behavioral sciences* (2nd ed.). Hillsdale, NJ: Lawrence Erlbaum Associates.

Cole, M. (1998). *Group dynamics in occupational therapy* (2nd ed.). Thorofare, NJ: Slack.

Corrigan, P. W., & Jakus, M. R. (1994). Behavioral treatment. In J. M. Silver, S. C. Yudofsky, & R. E. Hales (Eds.), *Neuropsychiatry of traumatic brain injury* (pp. 733-769). Washington, DC: American Psychiatric Press.

Corrigan, P. W., & McCracken, S. G. (1995). Refocusing the training of psychiatric rehabilitation staff. *Psychiatric Services, 46,* 1172-1177.

Csikszentmihalyi, M., & Csikszentmihalyi, I. S. (1988). *Optimal experience–Psychological studies of flow in consciousness.* New York: Cambridge University Press.

Custer, V. L., & Wassink, K. E. (1991). Occupational therapy intervention for an adult with depression and suicidal tendencies. *American Journal of Occupational Therapy, 45,* 845-848.

DeMarrias, K. D., & LeCompte, M. D. (1995). *The way schools work* (2nd ed., pp. 34-38). White Plains, NY: Longman.

Dickerson, A., & Oakley, F. (1995). Comparing the roles of community-living persons and patient populations. *American Journal of Occupational Therapy, 49,* 221-228.

Dickerson, F. B. (1997). Assessing clinical outcomes: The community functioning of persons with serious mental illness. *Psychiatric Services, 48,* 897-902.

Dion, G. L., & Anthony, W. A. (1987). Research in psychiatric rehabilitation: A review of experimental and quasi-experimental studies. *Rehabilitation Counseling Bulletin, 30,* 177-203.

Durkheim, E. (1938). *The rules of sociological method.* Chicago: The University of Chicago Press.

Durlak, J. A. (1998). Why program implementation is important. *Journal of Prevention & Intervention in the Community, 17,* 5-18.

Ebb, E., Coster, W., & Duncombe, L. (1989). Comparison of normal and psychosocially dysfunctional male adolescents. *Occupational Therapy in Mental Health, 9* (2), 53-74.

Endicott, J., Spitzer, R. L., Fleiss, J. L., & Cohen, J. (1976). The global assessment scale: A procedure for measuring overall severity of psychiatric disturbance. *Archives of General Psychiatry, 33,* 766-771.

Fidler, G. S. (1969). The task-oriented group as a context for treatment. *American Journal of Occupational Therapy, 32,* 305-310.

Fine, S. B. (1994). Reframing rehabilitation: Putting skill acquisition and the mental health system into proper perspective. In W. D. Spading (Ed.), *Cognitive technology in psychiatric rehabilitation* (pp. 87-113). Lincoln, NE: University of Nebraska Press.

Fleming, D., & Kaplan, J. P. (2000). Current and future public health challenges. *Journal of the American Medical Association, 284,* 1696-1698.

Frazier, R. S., & Baker-Smith, H. T. (1997). Predicting appropriate level of care in an innovative residential program design for people with mental illness. *Psychiatric Rehabilitation Journal, 21* (2), 181-184.

Geller, J. L., Fisher, W. H., McDermeit, M., & Brown, J. (1998). The effects of managed care on patterns of intensive use of inpatient psychiatric services. *Psychiatric Services, 49,* 327-332.

George, D., & Mallery, P. (2000). *SPSS for Windows step by step: A simple guide and reference 9.0 update* (2nd ed.). Boston: Allyn and Bacon.

George, L. K. (1993). Sociological perspectives on life transitions. *Annual Review of Sociology, 19,* 353-373.

Gillies, L. A., Wasylenki, D. A., Lancee, W. J., James, S., Clark, C. C., Lewis, J., & Goering, P. (1993). Differential outcomes in social network therapy. *Psychosocial Rehabilitation Journal, 16* (3), 141-146.

Goffman, E. (1961). *Asylums.* New York: Anchor Books.

Goldman, H. H., Skodol, A. E., & Lave, T. R. (1992). Revising Axis V for DSM-IV: A review of measures of social functioning. *American Journal of Psychiatry, 149,* 1148-1156.

Goldstein, A. P., Gershaw, N. J., & Sprafkin, R. P. (1979). Structured learning therapy: Development and evaluation. *American Journal of Occupational Therapy, 33,* 635-639.

Goodman, S. H., Sewell, D. R., Cooley, E. L., & Leavitt, N. (1993). Assessing levels of adaptive functioning: The role functioning scale. *Community Mental Health Journal, 29,* 119-131.

Gove, W., & Lubach, J. E. (1968). An intensive treatment program for psychiatric in-patients: A description and evaluation. *Journal of Health and Social Behavior, 9,* (4), 225-236.

Grace, G. R. (1972). *Role conflict and the teacher.* London: Routledge & Kegan Paul.

Green, R. S., & Gracely, E. J. Selecting a rating scale for evaluating services to the chronically mentally ill. *Community Mental Health Journal, 23,* 91-102.

Green, S. B., Salkind, N. J., & Akey, T. M. (2000). *Using SPSS for Windows: Analyzing and understanding data* (2nd ed.). Saddle River, NJ: Prentice-Hall.

Gross, N., Mason, W. S., & McEachern, A. W. (1958). *Explorations in role analysis.* New York: John Wiley and Sons.

Gutman, S. A. (1998). Alleviating gender role strain in adult men with traumatic brain injury: An assessment of a set of guidelines for occupational therapy. *American Journal of Occupational Therapy, 53,* 101-110.

Halford, W. K., Harrison, C., Kalyansundaram, Moutrey, C., & Simpson, S. (1995). Preliminary results from a psychoeducational program to rehabilitate chronic patients. *Psychiatric Services, 46,* 1189-1191.

Hardy, M. E., & Conway, M. E. (1978). *Role theory: Perspectives for health professionals.* New York: Appleton-Century-Crofts.

Heard, C. (1976). Occupational role acquisition: A perspective on the chronically disabled. *American Journal of Occupational Therapy, 31,* 243-247.

Heinssen, R. K., Liberman, R. P., & Kopelowicz, A. (2000). Psychosocial skills training for schizophrenia: Lessons from the laboratory. *Schizophrenia Bulletin, 26* (1), 21-46.

Heise, D. R., & Roberts, E. P. (1970). The development of role knowledge. *Genetic Psychology Monographs, 82,* 83-115.

Hocking, C. (2001). Implementing occupation-based assessment. *American Journal of Occupational Therapy, 55,* 463-469.

Howe, M. C., & Schwartzberg, S. L. (2001). *A functional approach to group work in occupational therapy* (3rd ed.). Philadelphia: Lippincott, Williams and Wilkins.

Jodrell, R. D., & Sanson-Fisher, R. (1975). Basic concepts of behavior therapy: An experiment involving disturbed adolescent girls. *American Journal of Occupational Therapy, 29,* 620-624.

Karmel, M. (1970). The internalization of social roles in institutionalized chronic mental patients. *Journal of Health and Social Behavior, 11* (9), 231-235.

Kauffman, J. M. (1996). Research to practice issues. *Behavioral Disorders, 22,* 55-60.

Kielhofner, G. (Ed.) (1985). *A model of human occupation.* Baltimore: Williams and Wilkins.

Kielhofner, G. (1995). *A model of human occupation* (2nd ed.). Baltimore: Williams and Wilkins.

Kielhofner, G. (2002). *Model of human occupation* (3rd ed.). Baltimore: Lippincott, Williams and Wilkins.

Kipper, D. A. (1991). The dynamics of role satisfaction: A theoretical model. *Journal of Group Psychotherapy, Psychodrama, and Sociometry, 44* (2), 71-86.

Labierte-Rudman, D., Yu, B., Scott, E., & Pajouhandeh, P. (2000). Exploration of the perspectives of persons with schizophrenia regarding quality of life. *American Journal of Occupational Therapy, 54,* 137-147.

Landy, R. J. (1991). The dramatic basis of role theory. *Arts in Psychotherapy, 18,* 29-41.

Law, M. (1998). Does client-centred practice make a difference? In M. Law (Ed.), *Client-centred occupational therapy.* Thorofare, NJ: Slack.

Law, M., Baptiste, S., & Mills, J. (1995). Client-centred practice: What does it mean and does it make a difference? *Canadian Journal of Occupational Therapy, 62,* 250-257.

Law, M., & Mills, J. (1998). Client-centred occupational therapy. In M. Law (Ed.), *Client-centred occupational therapy.* Thorofare, NJ: Slack.

Lededer, J. M., Kielhofner, G., & Watts, J. H. (1985). Values, personal causation and skills of delinquents and nondelinquents. *Occupational Therapy in Mental Health, 5* (2), 59-77.

Lehman, A. F. (1999). Quality of care in mental health: The case of schizophrenia. *Health Affairs, 18,* 52-65.

Lehman, A. F., & Steinwachs, D. M. (1998). At Issue: Translating research into practice: The schizophrenia patient outcomes research team (PORT) treatment recommendations. *Schizophrenia Bulletin, 24* (1), 1-10.

Levin, W. (1994). *Sociological ideas* (4th ed.). Belmont, CA: Wadsworth.

Liberman, R. P., & Kopelowicz, A. (2002). Teaching persons with severe mental disabilities to be their own case managers. *Psychiatric Services, 53* (11), 1377-1379.

Liberman, R. P., Wallace, C. J., Blackwell, G., Eckman, T. A., Vaccaro, J. V., & Kuehnel, T. G. (1993). Innovations in skills training for people with serious mental illness: The UCLA social and independent living skills modules. *Innovations & Research, 2* (2), 46-59.

Lillie, M. D., & Armstrong, H. E. (1982). Contributions to the development of psychoeducational approaches to mental health service. *American Journal of Occupational Therapy, 36,* 438-443.

Linton, R. (1936). *A study of man.* New York: Appleton-Century-Crofts.

Ludwig, E. G., & Adams, S. D. (1968). Patient cooperation in a rehabilitation center: Assumption of the client role. *Journal of Health and Social Behavior, 9* (4), 328-336.

Lyons, J. L., & Morse, A. R. (1988). A therapeutic work program for head-injured adults. *American Journal of Occupational Therapy, 42,* 364-370.

Mann, N. A., Tandon, R., Butler, J., Boyd, M., Eisner, W. H., & Lewis, M. (1993). Psychosocial rehabilitation in schizophrenia: Beginnings in acute hospitalization. *Archives of Psychiatric Nursing, 7,* 154-162.

Matsutsuyu, J. (1971). Occupational behavior–perspective on work and play. *American Journal of Occupational Therapy, 25,* 291-294.

Mattingly, C., & Fleming, M. H. (1994). *Clinical reasoning: Forms of inquiry in a therapeutic practice.* Philadelphia: F. A. Davis.

McGrew, J. H., Bond, G. R., Dietzen, L., & Salyers, M. (1994). Measuring the fidelity of implementation of a mental health program model. *Journal of Clinical and Consulting Psychology, 62,* 670-678.

McPheeters, H. L. (1984). Statewide mental health outcome evaluation: A perspective of two southern states. *Community Mental Health Journal, 20* (1), 44-55.

Mead, G. H. (1964). *On social psychology.* Chicago: The University of Chicago Press.

Mertler, C. A., & Vannatta, R. A. (2002). *Advanced and multivariate statistical methods.* 2nd ed. Los Angeles: Pyrczak Publishing.

Merton, R. K. (1957). *Social theory and social structure.* Chicago: The Free Press of Glencoe.

Miller, R. J. (1993). What is theory, and why does it matter? In R. J. Miller & K. F. Walker (eds.) *Perspectives on theory for the practice of occupational therapy.* Gaithersburg, MD: Aspen.

Mojtabai, R., Nicholson, R. A., & Carpenter, B. N. (1998). Role of psychosocial treatments in management of schizophrenia: A meta-analytic review of controlled outcome studies. *Schizophrenia Bulletin, 24,* 569-587.

Moncher, F. J., & Prinz, R. J. (1991). Treatment fidelity in outcome studies. *Clinical Psychology Review, 11,* 247-266.

Mosey, A. C. (1973). *Activities therapy.* New York: Raven Press.

Mosey, A. C. (1996). *Applied scientific inquiry in the health professions: An epistemological orientation* (2nd ed.). Bethesda, MD: American Occupational Therapy Association.

Mosey, A. C. (1986). *Psychosocial components of occupational therapy.* New York: Raven Press.

Mosey, A. C. (1970). *Three frames of reference for mental health.* Thorofare, NJ: Slack.

Oakley, F. (1981). *The role checklist.* Bethesda, MD: U. S. Department of Health and Human Services–National Institutes of Health.

Oakley, F., Kielhofner, G., & Barris, R. (1985). An occupational therapy approach to assessing psychiatric patients' adaptive functioning. *American Journal of Occupational Therapy, 39,* 147-154.

Oakley, F., Kielhofner, G., Barris, R., & Reichler, R. K. (1986). The role checklist: Development and empirical assessment of reliability. *Occupational Therapy Journal of Research, 6,* 157-170.

Parsons, T. (1951a). *The social system.* Glencoe, IL: The Free Press.

Parsons, T. (1951b). Illness and the role of the physician: A sociological perspective. *American Journal of Orthopsychiatry, 21,* 452-460.

Parsons, T., & Bales, R. (1955). *Family, socialization, and the interaction process.* New York: The Free Press of Glencoe.

Pearlin, L. I. (1983). Role strains and personal stress. In H. B. Kaplan (Ed.), *Psychosocial stress: Trends in theory and research* (pp. 3-33). New York: Academic Press.

Pollock, N., & McColl, M. (1998) Assessment in client-centred occupational therapy. In M. Law (Ed.) *Client-centred occupational therapy* (pp. 89-105). Thorofare, NJ: Slack.

Portnoy, L. G., & Watkins, M. P. (2000). *Foundations of clinical research: Applications to practice* (2nd ed.). Upper Saddle River, NJ: Prentice-Hall.

Posthuma, B. W. (1995). *Small groups in counseling and therapy: Process and leadership* (2nd ed). Toronto: Allyn and Bacon.

Reilly, M. (1962). Occupational therapy can be one of the great ideas of 20th Century medicine. *American Journal of Occupational Therapy, 16,* 1-9.

Reilly, M. (1969). The educational process. *American Journal of Occupational Therapy, 23,* 299-307.

Rice, K. G., & Meyer, A. L. (1994). Preventing depression among young adolescents: Preliminary process results of a psycho-educational intervention program. *Journal of Counseling and Development, 73,* 145-152.

Rogers, E. S., Sciarappa, K., & Anthony, W. A. (1991, Summer). Development and evaluation of situational assessment instruments and procedures for persons with psychiatric disabilities. *Vocational Evaluation and Work Adjustment Bulletin,* 61-67.

Ross, J. G., Leupler, R. V., Nelson, G. D., Saavedra, P., & Hubbard, B. M. (1991). Teenage health teaching modules: Impact of teacher training on implementation and student outcomes. *Journal of School Health, 61,* 31-34.

Ruddock, R. (1976). *Roles and relationships.* London: Routledge and Kegan Paul.

Sarbin, T. R. (1954). Role theory. In G. Lindzey (Ed.), *Handbook of social psychology* (pp. 223-258). Cambridge, MA: Addison-Wesley.

Sarbin, T. R., & Scheibe, K. E. (Eds.) (1983). *Studies in social identity.* New York: Praeger.

Sartorius, N. (1992). Rehabilitation and quality of life. *Psychiatric Services, 43,* 1180-1182.

Scanlon, J. W., Horst, P., Nay, J. N., Schmidt, R. E., & Waller, A. E. (1977). Evaluability assessment: Avoiding Type III and IV errors. In G. R. Gilbert & P. J. Conklin (Eds.), *Evaluation management: A source book of readings* (pp. 71-90). Charlottesville, VA: U. S. Civil Service Commission.

Schindler, V. (2002). The development of roles and role skills in adults diagnosed with schizophrenic disorders in a forensic setting. Ann Arbor, MI: UMI Dissertation Abstracts International.

Schindler, V., Connor, S. E., & Griffiths, S. (1995). The impact of a diverse psychiatric population on program development and training. *Conference Abstracts and Resources* (pp. 179-180). Bethesda, MD: American Occupational Therapy Association.

Schumacher, K. L. (1995). Family caregiver role acquisition: Role-making through situated interaction. *Scholarly Inquiry for Nursing Practice, 9,* 211-226.

Sepiol, J., & Froelich, J. (1990). Use of the role checklist with the patient with multiple personality disorder. *American Journal of Occupational Therapy, 44,* 1008-1012.

Shannon, P. D. (1972). Work-play theory and the occupational therapy process. *American Journal of Occupational Therapy, 26,* 169-172.

Sherry, L. (1997, March 5). Repeated measures and expected mean squares. Retrieved July 12, 2001, from http://carbon.cudenever.edu/~lsherry/rem/ems.html.

Slagle, E. C. (1924). A year's development of occupational therapy in New York State hospitals. *The Modern Hospital, 22,* 98-104.

Smith, A. R., & Tempone, V. J. (1968). Psychiatric occupational therapy within a learning theory context. *American Journal of Occupational Therapy, 22,* 415-425.

Smyntek, L., Barris, R., & Kielhofner, G. (1985). The Model of Human Occupation applied to psychosocially functional and dysfunctional adolescents. *Occupational Therapy in Mental Health, 5* (1), 21-39.

Sood, S., Baker, M., & Bledin, K. (1996). Social and living skills of new long-stay hospital patients and new long-term community patients. *Psychiatric Services, 47,* 619-622.

Stein, F., & Cutler, S. K. (1998). *Psychosocial occupational therapy: A holistic approach.* San Diego, CA: Singular.

Stephan, C. W., & Stephan, W. G. (1990). *Two social psychologies* (2nd ed.). Belmont, CA: Wadsworth Publishing.

Straube, E. R., & Oades, R. D. (1992). *Schizophrenia–Empirical research and findings.* New York: Academic Press.

Stuve, P., & Menditto, A. A. (1999). State hospitals in the new millennium: Rehabilitating the "Not ready for rehab players." *New Directions for Mental Health Services, 84,* 35-46.

Susser, M. W., Stein, Z., Mountey, G. H., & Freeman, H. L. (1970). Chronic disability following mental illness in an English city. Part I: Total prevalence in and out of mental hospital. *Social Psychiatry, 5,* 64-76.

Thoits, P. A. (1983). Multiple identities and psychological well-being: A reformulation and test of the social isolation hypothesis. *American Sociological Review, 48,* 174-187.

Trauer, T. (1998). Issues in the assessment of outcome in mental health. *Australian and New Zealand Journal of Psychiatry, 32,* 337-343.

Versluys, H. P. (1980). The remediation of role disorders through focused group work. *American Journal of Occupational Therapy, 34,* 609-614.

Wallace, C. J., Liberman, R. P., MacKain, S. J., Blackwell, G., & Eckman, T. A. (1992). Effectiveness and replicability of modules for teaching social and instrumental skills to the severely mentally ill. *American Journal of Psychiatry, 149,* 654-658.

Wanderer, Z. W. (1974). Therapy as learning: Behavior therapy. *American Journal of Occupational Therapy, 28,* 207-208.

Wapner, S., & Craig-Bray, L. (1992). Person-in-environment transitions: Theoretical and methodological approaches. *Environment and Behavior, 24,* 161-168.

Wessen, A. F. (1965). The apparatus of rehabilitation: An organizational analysis. In M. B. Sussman (Ed.), *Sociology and rehabilitation* (pp. 148-179). Washington, DC: American Sociological Association and the Vocational Rehabilitation Administration, US Department of Health, Education and Welfare.

Wing, J. K., Beevor, A. S., Curtis, R. H., Park, S. B., Hadden, S., & Burns, A. (1998). Health of the Nation Outcome Scale (HoNOS). *British Journal of Psychiatry, 172,* 11-18.

Wolfensberger, W. (2000). A brief overview of social role valorization. *Mental Retardation, 38,* 105-123.

World Health Organization (2001). *Classification of function, disability, and health.* Geneva, Switzerland: The Organisation.

APPENDICES

Appendix A:
Role Development Study Procedures

1. Receive the name and Role Checklist of a patient who is in the study and in your group.
2. Meet with the patient, orient him to your group, and conduct the Initial Staff/Patient Interview (located in the reference section of the manual). Use this time to select the activities and interactions the patient will have in the coming week.
3. Once you have an opportunity to observe and evaluate the patient, complete the appropriate Scales for your group (Task Skills Scale, Interpersonal Skills Scale, School, Work, Group Membership, and Friendships).
4. Complete Treatment Plan for the patient.
5. At least once a week, for 15 minutes, conduct the follow-up Staff/Patient Interview (located in the reference section of the manual). Use this time to select the activities and interactions the patient will have in the coming week.
6. Complete Progress Report for the week.
7. Continue meeting with the patient weekly until the patient completes the study (12 weeks) or is discharged from the hospital. Complete Progress Report after these meetings.
8. Complete the Fidelity Checklist (located in the reference section of the manual) when supervisor visits your group (approximately once every two weeks).

[Haworth co-indexing entry note]: "Appendix A: Role Development Study Procedures." Schindler, Victoria P. Co-published simultaneously in *Occupational Therapy in Mental Health* (The Haworth Press, Inc.) Vol. 20, No. 3/4, 2004, p. 163; and: *Occupational Therapy in Forensic Psychiatry: Role Development and Schizophrenia* (Victoria P. Schindler) The Haworth Press, Inc., 2004, p. 163. Single or multiple copies of this article are available for a fee from The Haworth Document Delivery Service [1-800-HAWORTH, 9:00 a.m. - 5:00 p.m. (EST). E-mail address: docdelivery@haworthpress.com].

http://www.haworthpress.com/web/OTMH
Digital Object Identifier: 10.1300/J004v20n03_12

Appendix B:
Role Development Initial Staff/Patient Interview
Role Development Rating Sheets
Role Development Treatment Plan
Progress Report

Role Development
Initial Staff/Patient Interview

Shortly after the patient begins in your group, spend about 15 minutes with him to get to know the roles and skills that will be appropriate for him to address (you will be given a copy of his completed Role Checklist). If you have not already done so, welcome him to your group, introduce him to the other members and give him a brief orientation to your group (e.g., the routine, the types of activities, rules for the group). Then ask him questions such as:

Your Role Checklist shows that you are interested in working on your (state all that apply to your group–friend, worker, student, group member) role (s). Did you have this role in the past? If so, what was it like for you? Can you tell me why you would like to work on this role now?

Do you have any ideas about how you would like to work on this role?

[Haworth co-indexing entry note]: "Appendix B: Role Development Initial Staff/Patient Interview, Role Development Rating Sheets, Role Development Treatment Plan, Progress Report." Schindler, Victoria P. Co-published simultaneously in *Occupational Therapy in Mental Health* (The Haworth Press, Inc.) Vol. 20, No. 3/4, 2004, pp. 165-175; and: *Occupational Therapy in Forensic Psychiatry: Role Development and Schizophrenia* (Victoria P. Schindler) The Haworth Press, Inc., 2004, pp. 165-175. Single or multiple copies of this article are available for a fee from The Haworth Document Delivery Service [1-800-HAWORTH, 9:00 a.m. - 5:00 p.m. (EST). E-mail address: docdelivery@haworthpress.com].

http://www.haworthpress.com/web/OTMH
© 2004 by The Haworth Press, Inc. All rights reserved.
Digital Object Identifier: 10.1300/J004v20n03_13

Give the patient some ideas about the way he can work on this role in your group (e.g., friend role–do an activity with another patient with whom he is comfortable). Would you like to do any of the suggestions this week?

Develop a plan with the patient of the activities and interactions he can attempt in the upcoming week.

Let the patient know that you will meet with him weekly to discuss his progress in working on the role.

1 Patient _____ Date _____ Staff _____

Task Skills

Task Behavior	Rating	Comments
1. Willingness to engage in doing tasks. Avoids engaging in tasks, talks more than engages in productive activity, needs prompting or encouragement to engage in task, seems fearful when engaging in tasks		
2. Physical capacity—includes posture, strength and gross and fine motor coordination. Is unable to assume and/or maintain a posture that is conducive to successful completion of the task, tires very easily and/or asks for or takes an inordinate number of rest periods, clumsy carrying out tasks and/or performs tasks very slowly because of need to concentrate on coordinated movements.		
3. Ability to maintain concentration on task. Short attention span, spends most of the time engaged in nontask-oriented behavior (e.g., walking around), frequently changes tasks, leaves tasks uncompleted.		
4. Ability to organize task in a logical manner. Appears not to think about task prior to beginning, does not have all the items needed for task completion close at hand, does not consider what should be done first, second, and so forth.		
5. Ability to follow directions. Unable to comprehend directions, unable to follow directions without assistance, repeatedly asks for directions when these have been given and/or when available, does not return to directions to check whether the task is being done correctly.		
6. Rate of performance. Unable to work at a steady pace, is excessively slow in performing a task so that little is accomplished in comparison to others, or is excessively fast so that quality is sacrificed, spends considerable time on tasks but is not productive.		
7. Attention to detail. Excessive attention to detail, is not certain what aspects of a task are more or less important, conversely there may be excessive disregard of details, hurries through tasks with little attention to details.		
8. Tolerates frustration. Becomes upset when confronted with a problem, has difficulty in accepting delays, becomes agitated when he or she makes a mistake, has difficulty in accepting negative feedback, does not like to repeat steps or to do something again.		

1 = Significantly below essential performance standards = Significantly fails to achieve standards defined for the group (e.g., does not work on the task, may show deviant or abusive behaviors toward the task).
2 = Below essential performance standards = Fails to meet standards defined for the group (e.g., needs assistance to productively engage in the task).
3 = Meets essential performance standards = Meets, but does not exceed, standards defined for the group (e.g., engages in the task as required or appropriate for the activity).
4 = Above essential performance standards = Exceeds standards defined for the group (e.g., readily and independently engages in task and exceeds level of performance required for task).
5 = Significantly above essential performance standards = Significantly exceeds standards defined for the group (e.g., can teach and supervise others in task completion, assistant to the group leader).
Additional Comments:

Note. From Psychosocial Components of Occupational Therapy (p. 322), by A. C. Mosey, 1986, New York: Raven Press. Copyright 1986 by Raven Press. Adapted with permission.

Patient _____ Date _____ Staff _____

Interpersonal Skills

Interpersonal Behavior	Rating	Comments
1. Ability to initiate, respond to, and sustain verbal interactions. Has difficulty in spontaneously initiating a conversation with another person, does not spontaneously respond to others, cannot carry on a conversation, is not able to participate in normal give-and-take of conversation.		
2. Keeps all statements appropriate to context. Cannot follow thread of discussion, makes statements that are inappropriate or irrelevant to subject matter, is unable to keep statements appropriate despite redirection.		
3. Communicates accurately and expresses self clearly. Does not communicate in a way that is sensible to the listener, communicates false statements, expresses ideas in a circuitous or tangential manner.		
4. Interacts comfortably with staff. Is overly shy, friendly or in need of constant attention from staff, is not able to request or receive assistance from staff, is not able to follow direction, rules, or procedures from staff.		
5. Interacts comfortably with peers. Is overly shy, aggressive, or inappropriate with peers, acts as though he or she has not considered the needs or feelings of others, is not able to work collaboratively with peers, is not able to accept help from peers.		
6. Uses appropriate non-verbal behavior and tone of voice. Invades the space of others, tone of voice and/or non-verbal gestures are inconsistent or inappropriate to verbal content or context of the situation.		
7. Cooperates as a member of a group. Avoids interacting in groups, acts independently in situations where cooperation is required, treats cooperative situations as if they were competitive, has difficulty being the winner or the loser in a competitive group situation.		
8. Controls impulsive, offensive, and/or annoying behavior. Hastily acts out toward self or others in a negative or harmful manner, intentionally irritates, torments, teases, or causes anguish to others, is verbally degrading or abusive to others.		

1 = Significantly below essential performance standards = Significantly fails to achieve standards defined for the group (e.g., does not interact with others, may show deviant or abusive behaviors toward others).
2 = Below essential performance standards = Fails to meet standards defined for the group (e.g., needs assistance for productive interaction with others).
3 = Meets essential performance standards = Meets, but does not exceed, standards defined for the group (e.g., engages in interaction as required or appropriate for the activity; is not disruptive to the group process).
4 = Above essential performance standards = Exceeds standards defined for the group (e.g., readily engages others in interactions, is helpful to others).
5 = Significantly above essential performance standards = Significantly exceeds standards defined for the group (e.g., assumes appropriate group leadership role, assistant to the group leader).
Additional Comments:

Note. From 1. *Psychosocial Components of Occupational Therapy* (p. 324), by A. C. Mosey, 1986, New York: Raven Press. Copyright 1986 by Raven Press. Adapted with permission. 2. Rogers, E. S., Sciarappa, K., & Anthony, W. A. (1991, Summer). Development and evaluation of situational assessment instruments and procedures for persons with psychiatric disabilities. *Vocational Evaluation and Work Adjustment Bulletin,* pp. 61-67.

Patient _____ Date _____ Staff _____

School

School Behavior	Rating	Comments
1. Class attendance. Frequently does not go to class, does not attend all classes, is late for and/or leaves early from class.		
2. Group behavior. Does not pay attention, disturbs other students, does not do tasks, does not participate in discussions.		
3. Relationship with teachers. Does not want to do what the teacher asks, ignores or is insolent to teacher, does not ask for guidelines or assistance when needed, cannot adapt to the style of some teachers, or is overly dependent on teacher.		
4. Relationship with classmates. States that he or she has no friends in class, is excessively shy with classmates, is a loner, or provokes classmates, acts as if superior to others, is not liked by classmates.		
5. Academic performance. Grades are below what one would expect given the individual's apparent abilities, grades are markedly uneven across subjects and/or grading periods, does not seem to put forth much effort, blames poor academic performance on others.		
6. Participation in academic evaluations. Does not study adequately for tests, hurries through examinations without giving appropriate attention to each item, or becomes excessively anxious prior to or during test, is overly preoccupied with grades.		

1 = Significantly below essential performance standards = Significantly fails to achieve standards defined for school (e.g., does not work on the task, may show deviant or abusive behaviors toward the task).
2 = Below essential performance standards = Fails to meet standards defined for school (e.g., needs assistance to productively engage in the task).
3 = Meets essential performance standards = Meets, but does not exceed, standards defined for school (e.g., engages in the task as required or appropriate for the assignment).
4 = Above essential performance standards = Exceeds standards defined for school (e.g., readily and independently engages in the task and exceeds level of performance required for the task).
5 = Significantly above essential performance standards = Significantly exceeds standards defined for school (e.g., can teach and supervise others in task completion, assistant to the teacher).
Additional Comments:

Note. From *Psychosocial Components of Occupational Therapy* (p. 322), by A. C. Mosey, 1986, New York: Raven Press. Copyright 1986 by Raven Press. Adapted with permission. V. Schindler, PhD, OTR, 2002.

169

Patient _____ Date _____ Staff _____

Work

Work Behavior	Rating	Comments
1. Attendance. Attendance at work is irregular, frequently late to work, leaves work early, has difficulty tolerating a full session of work.		
2. General attitude. Does not feel the role of worker is an important social role, does not see self as a worker, is happier when not working.		
3. Performance. Manifests fear or anxiety as a response to the demand to be productive, does not organize tasks relative to priority, does not work at increased speeds when required, does not easily return to work after interruptions, does not plan work periods so that required amount of work is accomplished, avoids responsibility, does not complete assigned tasks in an acceptable manner, completes assigned tasks late.		
4. Take direction from work supervisor. Acts in a hostile or aggressive manner when assigned work, does not follow directions given, unable to accept constructive criticism, or is overly dependent on supervisor.		
5. Relationship to co-workers. Is overly dependent, does not give assistance when requested, is unable to carry on a casual conversation with co-workers, responds to co-workers in a belligerent manner, makes derogatory remarks to co-workers, avoids co-workers during breaks and lunch hour, acts in a way that makes co-workers uncomfortable.		
6. Response to norms of the work setting. Does not dress appropriately, selects inappropriate topics of conversation, pace of work is markedly different from workers, acts as if the work setting is designed to suit needs that are more appropriately satisfied in other settings, does not conform to the rules of the setting, cannot differentiate between formal and informal structure.		

1 = Significantly below essential performance standards = Significantly fails to achieve standards defined for work (e.g., does not work on the task, may show deviant or abusive behaviors toward the task).
2 = Below essential performance standards = Fails to meet standards defined for work (e.g., needs assistance to productively engage in the task).
3 = Meets essential performance standards = Meets, but does not exceed, standards defined for work (e.g., engages in the task as required or appropriate for the activity).
4 = Above essential performance standards = Exceeds standards defined for work (e.g., readily and independently engages in task and exceeds level of performance required for the task).
5 = Significantly above essential performance standards = Significantly exceeds standards defined for the group (e.g., can teach and supervise others in task completion, assistant to the group leader).
Additional Comments:

Note. From *Psychosocial Components of Occupational Therapy* (p. 322), by A. C. Mosey, 1986, New York: Raven Press. Copyright 1986 by Raven Press. Adapted with permission. V. Schindler, PhD, OTR, 2002.

Patient _____ Date _____ Staff _____

Group Membership

Group Membership Behavior	Rating	Comments
1. Group attendance. Frequently does not go to group, does not attend all group sessions, is late for and/or leaves early from group sessions.		
2. Group behavior. Does not pay attention, disturbs other group members, does not do tasks, does not participate in discussions.		
3. Relationship with group leaders. Does not want to do what the group leader asks, ignores or is insolent to group leader, does not ask for guidelines or assistance when needed, cannot adapt to the style of some group leaders, or, is overly dependent on group leader.		
4. Relationship with group members. States that he or she has no friends in group, is excessively shy, avoids others during breaks, is unable to carry on a casual conversation, does not give assistance when requested, responds to others in a belligerent manner, makes derogatory remarks, acts as if superior to others, is not liked by group members.		
5. Performance. Manifests fear or anxiety as a response to the demand to be productive, does not organize tasks relative to priority, does not work at increased speeds when required, does not easily return to work after interruptions, does not plan work periods so that required amount of work is accomplished, avoids responsibility, does not complete assigned tasks in an acceptable manner, completes assigned tasks late.		
6. Response to norms of the setting. Does not dress appropriately, selects inappropriate topics of conversation, pace of task completion is markedly different from peers, does not conform to the rules of the setting.		

1 = **Significantly below essential performance standards** = Significantly fails to achieve standards defined for the group (e.g., does not work on the task, may show deviant or abusive behaviors toward the task).
2 = **Below essential performance standards** = Fails to meet standards defined for the group (e.g., needs assistance to productively engage in the task).
3 = **Meets essential performance standards** = Meets, but does not exceed, standards defined for the group (e.g., engages in the task as required or appropriate for the activity).
4 = **Above essential performance standards** = Exceeds standards defined for the group (e.g., readily and independently engages in the task and exceeds level of performance required for the task).
5 = **Significantly above essential performance standards** = Significantly exceeds standards defined for the group (e.g., can teach and supervise others in task completion, assistant to the group leader).
Additional Comments:

Note. From *Psychosocial Components of Occupational Therapy* (p. 322), by A. C. Mosey, 1986, New York: Raven Press. Copyright 1986 by Raven Press. Adapted with permission. V. Schindler, PhD, OTR, 2002.

Patient _____ Date _____ Staff _____

Friendships

Friendship Behavior	Rating	Comments
1. Initiates friendships. States that he or she has no friends, does not know how to go about establishing friend relationships, states that there is no one that he or she can talk to.		
2. Maintains friendships. Spends little if any time with other people outside of the context of school/work/ groups, has friendships for only a short period of time.		

1 = **Significantly below essential performance standards** = Significantly fails to achieve standards defined for the group (e.g., does not interact with others, may show deviant or abusive behaviors toward others).

2 = **Below essential performance standards** = Fails to meet standards defined for the group (e.g., needs assistance for productive interaction with others).

3 = **Meets essential performance standards** = Meets, but does not exceed, standards defined for the group (e.g., engages in interaction as required or appropriate for the activity; is not disruptive to the group process).

4 = **Above essential performance standards** = Exceeds standards defined for the group (e.g., readily engages others in interactions, is helpful to others).

5 = **Significantly above essential performance standards** = Significantly exceeds standards defined for the group (e.g., assumes appropriate group leadership role, assistant to the group leader).
Additional Comments:

Note. From *Psychosocial Components of Occupational Therapy* (p. 322), by A. C. Mosey, 1986, New York: Raven Press. Copyright 1986 by Raven Press. Adapted with permission. V. Schindler, PhD, OTR, 2002.

Role Development – Treatment Plan

Staff Name _____ Date _____
Patient Name _____

1. Of the following roles (worker, student, friend, group member), which role(s) would you identify as being relevant for this patient? Why?

2. Evaluate the patient's skills by completing the Task Skills Scale and the Interpersonal Skills Scale and any other appropriate scales (i.e., school, work, group membership, friendship).

3. Identify and prioritize the skill and role areas that need to be addressed.

Task Skills	Interpersonal Skills	Role _____	Role _____
a. _____	a. _____	a. _____	a. _____
b. _____	b. _____	b. _____	b. _____
c. _____	c. _____	c. _____	c. _____

4. Read the corresponding Methods to Promote Positive Change and list 1 or more ideas and activities/interventions to promote change for each deficient skill or role.

Deficient Skill –Task	Idea to Promote Change	Activity/Intervention

Deficient Skill – Interpersonal	Idea to Promote Change	Activity/Intervention

Deficient Role_____	Idea to Promote Change	Activity/Intervention
Deficient Role_____	Idea to Promote Change	Activity/Intervention
Deficient Role_____	Idea to Promote Change	Activity/Intervention
Deficient Role_____	Idea to Promote Change	Activity/Intervention

Progress Report

Staff Name _____   Date _____
Patient Name _____
Week _____

Task Skills	___Progress ___NO Progress Rationale:	Plan for next week
Interpersonal Skills	___Progress ___NO Progress Rationale:	Plan for next week
Role _____	___Progress ___NO Progress Rationale:	Plan for next week
Role _____	___Progress ___NO Progress Rationale:	Plan for next week
Deficient Skill – Other	Idea to Promote Change	Activity/Intervention
Deficient Skill – Other	Idea to Promote Change	Activity/Intervention

Index

Action-Consequence frame of
      reference, 20-21
Activities Therapy, 20-21
Administrative implications, 146
Affective flattening, 16
Alogia, 16
Alpha coefficients, of pilot study,
      69-70
ANOVA
      differences over time, 138
      Role Development, 137
Attention to detail, 39
Atypical/typical development, 29-30
Avolition, 16

Behavior, impulse control, 41-42
Behavioral indicators, of
      function/dysfunction, 30-34
Box's Test of Equality of Covariance
      Measures, 90-91, 98

Case studies, 111-122
Catatonic motor behaviors, 16
Clinical supervision, 55
Cognitive skills, 20
Collaborative, client-centered
      approach, 141-142
Communication/self-expression, 40
Comparison group, 61-62
      analysis of qualitative findings, 108
      individual attention in, 98-100
      patient interviews, 106-107
      pilot study, 73
      pretest results, 83
Concentration ability, 37-38

Context-appropriateness, 40
Correlation coefficients, 96-100

Data analysis, 75-77
Delusions, 15
Demographics, staff, 123-124
Detail, attention to, 39
Development, typical/atypical, 29-30
Directions, ability to follow, 38
Disorganized thinking, 16
DSM-IV, 4,58,59,82
Dysfunctional roles, 4-5

Effectiveness. *See also* Qualitative
      evaluation; Quantitative
      evaluation
      qualitative evaluation, 105-109
      quantitative data, 79-104
Experimental group, 62-63
      analysis of qualitative findings, 108
      patient interviews, 107-108
      pilot study, 74-76
      pretest results, 84-85

Fidelity
      ongoing, 55-56
      treatment, 52-55
Fidelity Checklist, 56
      principal investigator, 125-126
      staff, 125
Findings, 133-149
      conclusions, 148-149
      implications of study, 139-140,
            144-146

interpersonal skills, 135-136
limitations of study, 146-148
Role Development, 136-137
success-promoting attributes,
140-144
task skills, 134-135
time/skill development relationship,
137-139
Focus groups, staff, 77, 126-132
Following directions, 38
Friendships
function/dysfunction continuums, 34
interview checklist, 172
postulates for positive change, 36,
44-45
Frustration, tolerance for, 39
Function/dysfunction continuums,
26-27,30,31-34
friendships, 34
group membership, 34
interpersonal skills, 32
school roles, 32-33
task skills, 31
work roles, 33

Generalizability issues, 146
Global Assessment Functioning Scale,
58-59
Group cooperation, 41
Group membership, 13-14
function/dysfunction continuums,
34
interview checklist, 171
postulates for positive change, 36,44

Hallucinations, 15-16
Hospitalization, isolation and, 17
Hypotheses of study, 7

Implementation
by staff, 50-52
treatment fidelity, 52-55

Implementation tools, 47-56
staff training, 47-50
Implications, 139-140
administrative, 146
for client population, 139
research, 148
for staff, 144-146
Impulse control, 41-42
Individuality, 27, 70
Instruments. *See also individual
measures*
Global Assessment Functioning
Scale, 58-59
Interpersonal Skills Scale, 68
inter-rater reliability, 147
Role Checklist, 66-68
Role Functioning Scale, 64-66
Task Skills Scale, 68
Internal validity, 147
Interpersonal skills, 18-20
findings, 135-136
function/dysfunction continuums,
32
interview checklist, 168
postulates for positive change, 36,
39-42
Interpersonal Skills Scale, 7, 68
inter-rater reliability, 70-71, 147
quantitative evaluation, 86-87
relationship of scales, 96-100
repeated-measures ANOVA, 93-96
Inter-rater reliability, of pilot study,
70-71
Interviews
initial, 164-165
patient, 106-109

JCAHO accreditation, 146

Learning, Principles of, 29
Learning objectives, 27-28
Learning process, 28-29
Limitations of study, 146-148

instrumentation, 147
staff, 147

MANCOVA, 96-98
    interpersonal skills, 135-136
    Role Development, 137
    task skills effectiveness, 134-135
Maximum-security settings, 5-7. *See
    also* Role Development
Meaningful occupation, as
        success-promoting attribute,
        142-143
Method. *See* Outcomes-based study
Motor behaviors, catatonic, 16
Multiple roles, 14

Nonverbal behavior, postulates for
        change, 41

Occupational Behavior frame of
        reference, 21
Organizational ability, 38
Outcomes-based study, 57-77. *See also*
        Instruments
    comparison group, 61-62
    data analysis, 75-77
    design, 60-63
    experimental group, 62-63
    instrumentation, 63-68
    pilot study, 69-75. *See also* Pilot
        study
    recruitment, 59-60
    sample, 57-59
    staff focus groups, 77
    staff participants, 60

Patient interviews, 106-109,164-165
Peer interactions, 40
Performance rate, 38
Physical capacity, for tasks, 37
Pilot study, 69-75
    alpha coefficients, 69-70

experimental group, 74-76
    fidelity, 75
    inter-rater reliability, 70-71
    pretest/posttest evaluation
        procedure, 72
    recruitment, 73
    staff training, 73-74
Post-study staff focus groups, 128-132
Postulates for positive change, 27,
        35-46
    communication/self-expression, 40
    context-appropriateness, 40
    friendships, 36, 44-45
    general, 35
    group cooperation, 41
    group membership, 33,36,44
    impulse control, 41-42
    interpersonal skills, 36, 39-42
    nonverbal behavior, 41
    peer interactions, 40
    school, 36, 42
    specific, 36-46
    staff interactions, 40
    task skills, 36, 37-39
    verbal interaction capability, 39
    work, 36, 42-44
Practice guidelines, 35-45
    behavioral indicators of
        function/dysfunction, 30-34
    fidelity to, 55-56
    function/dysfunction continuums,
        26-27,30,31-34
    postulates to promote positive
        change, 35-45
    staff instruction in, 45-46
    as success-promoting attributes,
        140-144
    theoretical base, 26,27-30
Pretest/posttest evaluation procedure, 72
Pretest results
    comparison group, 83
    experimental group, 84-85
Pre-training staff focus groups, 126-128
Principles of Learning, 29
Problem statement, 7
Program drift, 52

Qualitative evaluation, 105-109
    conclusion, 109
    patient interviews, 106-109
Quality of life, 143-144
Quantitative evaluation, 79-104
    conclusion, 103-104
    Interpersonal Skills Scale, 86-87
    interscale relationships, 96-100
    MANCOVA, 84-85
    patient demographics, 79-84
    pretest results, 82-84
    repeated-measures ANOVA, 89-95
    Role Checklist, 100-103
    Role Functioning Scale, 87-89
    Task Skills Scale, 85-86

Rate of performance, 38-39
Recruitment, 59-60
References, 151-159
Repeated-measures ANOVA, 89-95
    Interpersonal Skills Scale, 93-96
    Role Functioning Scale, 91-92
    Task Skills Scale, 92-93
Research implications, 148
Role Acquisition, 5-6,20-22
Role Checklist
    inter-rater reliability, 70-71
    quantitative evaluation, 100-103
Role Development, 5,11-23
    case studies, 111-122
    conclusion, 22-23
    findings, 136-137
    implementation tools, 47-56
    participating staff, 123-126
    practice guidelines, 20-22
    progress report, 185
    qualitative evaluation, 105-109
    quantitative evaluation, 79-104
    in schizophrenic disorders, 15-18
    skills development and, 18-20
    staff response, 123-133
    treatment guidelines, 25-45, See
        also Practice guidelines
    treatment plan, 173-174

Role Functioning Scale, 7,19
    inter-rater reliability, 70-71
    quantitative evaluation, 87-89
    relationship of scales, 96-100
    repeated-measures ANOVA, 91-92
Role theory, 11-15
    group aspects, 13-14
    multiple roles, 14
    Social Role Valorization, 14-15
    structural functionalism, 12-13
    symbolic interactionism, 12-13
    variance within roles, 13

Schizophrenia
    clinical features, 15-16
    negative symptoms, 16
    positive symptoms, 16
    sick role in, 16-17
    social network theory, 17-18
School
    function/dysfunction continuums, 32
    interview checklist, 169
    postulates for positive change, 36,
        42
Sick role, 16-17
Skill development, 18-20
Social network theory, 17-18
Social roles. See also Role entries
    defined, 2-3
    development of, 3. See also Role
        Development
    dysfunctional, 4-5
    hypotheses, 7
    interpersonal skills and, 3-4, See
        also Interpersonal skills; Skill
        development
    maximum-security settings and, 5-7
    mental illness and, 4
    problem statement, 7
    schizophrenia and, 1-10
Social Role Valorization, 14-15
Spearman correlation coefficients,
    96-100
Staff

compliance data, 125-126
conclusion, 132
demographics, 123-124
implications of study for, 144-146
Staff focus groups, 77,126-132
post-study, 128-132
pre-training, 126-128
Staff interactions, 40
Staff interview, 164-165
Staff response, 123-133
Staff study participants, 60
Staff training, 47-50
assessment, 48
didactic instruction on practice
guidelines, 48-49
group and individual case studies,
49-50
homework/posttest assignment, 50
individual, 50
pilot study, 73-74
simulations, 49
Structural functionalism, 12-13
Study design. *See* Outcomes-based
study
Study procedures, 163
Success-promoting attributes, 140-144
collaborative, client-centered
approach, 141-142
meaningful occupation, 142-143
practice guidelines, 140-141
quality of life, 143-144
Supervision, of staff, 54-55
Symbolic interactionism, 12-13

Task skills, 18-20
findings, 134-135
function/dysfunction continuums,
31

interview checklist, 167
postulates for positive change, 36,
37-39
Task Skills Scale, 7,68
inter-rater reliability, 70-71, 147
quantitative evaluation, 85-86
relationship of scales, 96-100
repeated-measures ANOVA, 92-93
Theoretical base, of practice
guidelines, 26,27-30
Time/skill development relationship,
137-139
Tolerance for frustration, 39
Tools, for performance evaluation, 30.
See also Instruments
Training. *See* Staff training
Treatment differentiation, 53
Treatment fidelity, 52-56
Treatment guidelines, 35-45. *See also*
Practice guidelines
Treatment manuals, 54
Treatment plan, 173-174
Typical/atypical development, 29-30

Validity, internal, 147
Verbal interaction capability, 39

Willingness, for tasks, 37
Work
function/dysfunction continuums,
33
interview checklist, 170
postulates for positive change, 36,
42-44

BOOK ORDER FORM!

Order a copy of this book with this form or online at:
http://www.haworthpress.com/store/product.asp?sku=5350

Occupational Therapy in Forensic Psychiatry
Role Development and Schizophrenia

_____ in softbound at $19.95 (ISBN: 0-7890-2125-0)
_____ in hardbound at $34.95 (ISBN: 0-7890-2124-2)

COST OF BOOKS _____

POSTAGE & HANDLING _____
US: $4.00 for first book & $1.50
for each additional book
Outside US: $5.00 for first book
& $2.00 for each additional book.

SUBTOTAL _____

In Canada: add 7% GST. _____

STATE TAX _____
CA, IL, IN, MN, NJ, NY, OH & SD residents
please add appropriate local sales tax.

FINAL TOTAL _____
If paying in Canadian funds, convert
using the current exchange rate.
UNESCO coupons welcome.

❏ BILL ME LATER:
Bill-me option is good on US/Canada/
Mexico orders only; not good to jobbers,
wholesalers, or subscription agencies.

❏ Signature _____

❏ Payment Enclosed: $ _____

❏ PLEASE CHARGE TO MY CREDIT CARD:
❏ Visa ❏ MasterCard ❏ AmEx ❏ Discover
❏ Diner's Club ❏ Eurocard ❏ JCB

Account # _____

Exp Date _____

Signature _____
(Prices in US dollars and subject to change without notice.)

PLEASE PRINT ALL INFORMATION OR ATTACH YOUR BUSINESS CARD

Name		
Address		
City	State/Province	Zip/Postal Code
Country		
Tel	Fax	
E-Mail		

May we use your e-mail address for confirmations and other types of information? ❏ Yes ❏ No We appreciate receiving
your e-mail address. Haworth would like to e-mail special discount offers to you, as a preferred customer.
We will never share, rent, or exchange your e-mail address. We regard such actions as an invasion of your privacy.

Order From Your **Local Bookstore** or Directly From
The Haworth Press, Inc. 10 Alice Street, Binghamton, New York 13904-1580 • USA
Call Our toll-free number (1-800-429-6784) / Outside US/Canada: (607) 722-5857
Fax: 1-800-895-0582 / Outside US/Canada: (607) 771-0012
E-mail your order to us: orders@haworthpress.com

For orders outside US and Canada, you may wish to order through your local
sales representative, distributor, or bookseller.
For information, see http://haworthpress.com/distributors

(Discounts are available for individual orders in US and Canada only, not booksellers/distributors.)

Please photocopy this form for your personal use.
www.HaworthPress.com

BOF04

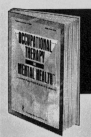
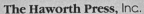